"The ancient practice of yoga  era as a valuable method fo being. *Yoga Mind, Peaceful Mi* rewarding practice, and can add serenity, joy, and ... ment to your life."

—**Larry Dossey, MD**, author of *One Mind*

"*Yoga Mind, Peaceful Mind* is a wonderful resource for those choosing to take the yogic path to address issues related to anxiety, depression, and trauma. The information provided on the chakras is especially useful to survivors of trauma, and the practical meditations on each chakra will help survivors to realize the power of this content."

—**Jamie Marich, PhD**, creator of Dancing Mindfulness and author of *Trauma and the Twelve Steps*, *Trauma Made Simple*, and *EMDR Made Simple*

"This book connects the reader in a direct experiential way with the teachings of the great Eastern wisdom traditions on how to obtain peace of mind by accessing inner strength through simple, beautiful yoga and meditation. The book achieves its goals without using too many words and by adopting a language that is direct and personal as well as easy to understand and follow. The authors do not attempt to convince but instead constantly encourage readers to open up to and tap into their energy centers (chakras) to experience for themselves the vast inner resources and richness we have all been blessed with."

—**Georg H. Eifert, PhD**, emeritus professor of psychology at Chapman University in Orange, CA, and coauthor of *The Mindfulness and Acceptance Workbook for Anxiety*

"For many of us in the 21st century, life feels hectic and stressful. To make matters worse, many Americans are wandering around in what Tara Brach refers to as 'a trance of unworthiness,' having forgotten the radiant quality of our own true nature. In *Yoga Mind, Peaceful Mind*, Mary and Rick NurrieStearns present accessible practices to discover your true nature and to train your mind to be a powerful instrument for happiness and peace—in your life and in the lives of those around you. Moreover, the authors offer a skilled account of our chakra system from the ancient wisdom of the yoga tradition. If you are interested in enlivening your mind, body, and energy, you should read this book."

—**Terry Fralich**, counselor, attorney, teacher, and author of *The Five Core Skills of Mindfulness*

"Anxiety is a cognitive echo of fear. All fear is based on the illusory duality of self and other. Whereas fear divides, yoga unites. Yoga-mind erases the distinction between self and other and, in so doing, unifies the I-figure with the ground of All That Is. This isn't Buddhist psychology. This is Vedic psychology. There is a difference. Buddhist psychology works by helping you see through the illusion of the ego-based self and stops there. Vedic psychology goes a step further: in shedding the illusion of this separate, fearful self, it introduces you to your true, essential Self, to the kind of Self that is united with All That Is, and thus knows no fear. The NurrieStearnses' book is an excellent invitation to a reunion with your own fearlessness."

—**Pavel Somov, PhD**, author of *The Lotus Effect*

"*Yoga Mind, Peaceful Mind* provides inviting meditative experiences guiding readers to healthy being. The authors sensitively integrate chakra wisdom with useful psychological teachings for healing from root to crown. With depth and beauty, simple yet profound, many will find a clear path to inner peace."

—**Annellen Simpkins, PhD, and C. Alexander Simpkins, PhD**, workshop leaders and authors of 28 books, including *The Tao of Bipolar, Neuroscience for Clinicians*, and *Yoga and Mindfulness Therapy Workbook*

yoga mind, peaceful mind

---

simple meditations for
overcoming anxiety

Mary NurrieStearns
Rick NurrieStearns

New Harbinger Publications, Inc.

Publisher's Note

This publication is designed to provide accurate and authoritative information in regard to the subject matter covered. It is sold with the understanding that the publisher is not engaged in rendering psychological, financial, legal, or other professional services. If expert assistance or counseling is needed, the services of a competent professional should be sought.

Distributed in Canada by Raincoast Books

Copyright © 2015 by Mary NurrieStearns and Rick NurrieStearns
New Harbinger Publications, Inc.
5674 Shattuck Avenue
Oakland, CA 94609
www.newharbinger.com

Cover design by Amy Shoup; Interior design by Michele Waters-Kermes; Acquired by Jess O'Brien; Edited by Elizabeth Berg

Chakras and Chakra Woman Illustrations © Peter Hermes Furian | Dreamstime.com

Library of Congress Cataloging-in-Publication Data on file

56563900 4/15

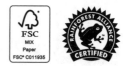

Printed in the United States of America

17   16   15

10   9   8   7   6   5   4   3   2   1   First printing

Contents

Acknowledgments

We are grateful to all who contributed to making this book a reality. A heartfelt thank-you goes to New Harbinger Publications, who backed us all the way from idea to printing. We give special thanks to Jess O'Brien, who guided the book concept and design and made this book possible. A thank-you also goes to Jess Beebe for waving her mighty wand of focus and consistency over the chapters and to Elizabeth Berg for expert copyediting.

We thank Ellie Finlay, whose feedback added depth and clarity. We are grateful to the yogis who have passed down knowledge about the chakras and healing, especially Swami Saraswati, Swami Saradananda, Swami Rama, and Anodea Judith, whose works informed and inspired this book.

A loving bow of appreciation goes to our retreatants and yoga students for embracing the healing practices of yoga and verifying again and again the transformative power of ongoing practice. Your love touches us deeply, sustains us more than you know, and keeps us faithful to our practice and study.

With hands at our hearts, we express gratitude to family, pets, and friends for loving us and hanging in there through thick and thin. Love and appreciation go to Thich Nhat Hahn and Father Thomas Keating for guidance on the spiritual path. We honor Maurice Hoover for encouraging us to write mindfully, Sara Alavi for believing in our work, and Meghan Donnally for providing a yoga studio home for us.

And now, dear reader, thank you. This book is for you. You were in our hearts throughout the year of writing. Your willingness to embrace yoga to reduce suffering and increase happiness makes us kindred spirits. May these pages contribute to your well-being.

Introduction

Your remarkable mind has many capacities: it thinks, develops a personal identity, makes decisions, coordinates actions, remembers, and acts instinctually to keep you safe. You can also train your mind to be an instrument of peace. Yogic discplines show you how. They help you to understand how your mind works, as well as how to witness thoughts and concentrate on what matters most. As a result of practicing yoga, your anxiety lessens and your mind helps you fulfill your life's purpose.

Your mind encompasses much more than the brain, that incredible organ in your skull. It is spread throughout your physical body via the nervous system that runs along the spine and out into your torso and limbs. Neuroscientist Daniel Siegel (2010) defines the mind as a relationship process embodied in the physical body that regulates the flow of information and energy in the brain. However you define it, your mind is a process, not a body part, that has amazing abilities. It takes in information and energy, decides how to respond to incoming data, and fundamentally is your instrument of thinking, sensing, and consciousness.

Neuroscientists define the mind in ways that parallel how yogis describe the chakras. Ancient yogis understood that your chakra system pertains to consciousness, lacks finite boundaries, and manages your life energy. They characterized the chakra system as a series of spinning wheels composed of energy and consciousness that run along or just in front of the spine, from your tailbone through your brain to above the crown of your head. There is a fundamental difference between how the yogis conceived of chakras and how scientists conceive of the mind. Scientists do not include higher consciousness in their definition of the mind. In the chakra system, consciousness begins with basic physical survival, moves up through concerns of the human heart, and reaches beyond to include understanding of the spiritual oneness of life. In fact, the primary goals of yoga are to help you become aware of your mind, discover you are a conscious being having a human experience, and train your mind to serve the sacred unity of life.

According to Anodea Judith (2010), chakras are centers where life-force energy is received, assimilated, and expressed. Although aligned along the spine, they are states of consciousness rather than distinct physical matter. They exist at the meeting place of matter and spirit, and each center uniquely contributes to your health, emotional stability, and spiritual awareness.

Chakras have no finite boundaries and are highly sensitive. Whatever goes on in the world around you affects your chakras, especially the inevitable traumas and difficulties that block your chakras. What transpires inside you, such as painful emotions, also affects your chakras. Blockages negatively affect your sense of identity, the quality of your emotional life, what you value, and how you experience life.

Working with the chakras clears away blockages. However, these blockages deserve utmost respect because they began as defensive patterns to protect your innermost self and then became unconscious and stuck. The meditations in this book are keys that unlock the blockages and give you a yoga mind—one that focuses on love and the truth that you are a spiritual being interconnected with all life.

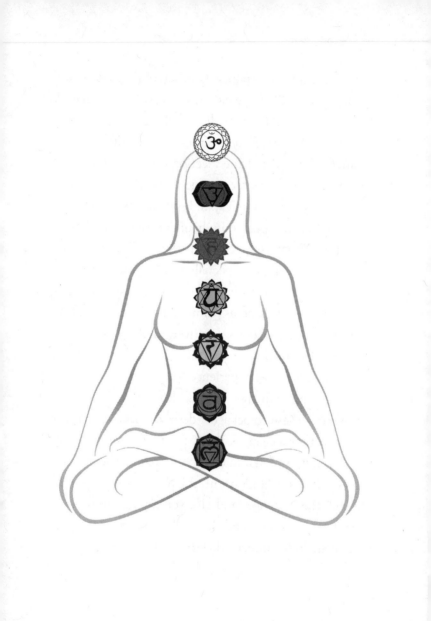

chapter 1

True Self, False Self

The most painful cause of anxiety is probably the belief that you are not enough. This belief, when deeply buried and unseen, often takes the form of painstaking efforts to improve who you are—attempts that frequently result in inner exhaustion and discontentment. You may do honorable work and make a positive difference and still feel plagued by feelings of inadequacy. Trying to make yourself worthy is ineffective and misses the mark. You cannot make yourself into something you already are.

The way out of this mental trap is not by positive affirmations, although wise words can point to the truth. The way out is realizing who you truly are. The way out is comforting yourself for how much you have suffered because you did not know your true identity as a spiritual being.

Yoga philosophy teaches that you have two coexisting identities, one true and one false. Your true self is with you at birth, long before you understand language and the power of words. Your false self depends upon language and reflects your ideas about who you are. Your false self, or "made-up" identity, consists of self-limiting beliefs that tear you down, causing you to feel inferior to others, and grandiose beliefs that prop you up to make you feel superior to others. Your true self, or spiritual self, is the aware presence within you that naturally experiences clarity, inner peace, love, and a sense of connectedness not based on thoughts or mental outlook. As a spiritual being, you do not need a story to be somebody, and yet, as a human being, you also have a story line about who you are.

You have some awareness of your false identity. It is how you define yourself in words and images. Developing a false identity, *ahankara,* or sense of *I-ness* (Rama, Ballentine, and Ajaya 1976), is natural and inevitable. It is your personal narrative about the kind of person you are, derived from what happened or did not happen to you, what others said or did not say, what you believe and do not believe about who you are.

You may or may not be aware of your true self, or *Parusha*, consciousness itself (Rama, Ballentine, and Ajaya 1976), which is easier to notice when your mind is quiet. You have probably experienced a sense of profound inner stillness during moments of prayer and meditation or in the stillness of the wilderness. During such moments, you experienced your inner self, whether or not you recognized this as your true self.

This chapter, focused on a practice of *svadhyaya* (a Sanskrit word meaning "study of the self"), will help you lovingly accept who you think you are and realize who you truly are. The following meditations will help you experience your true self and gently release the grip of your false self. They will teach you to recognize your made-up self-identity so that you can say, "Wait a minute, I just fell into the old story of who I am," turn your attention to your innermost self, and experience the heartfelt relief found there.

The main message of this chapter is that all life, including yours, is sacred. You are worthy because you are.

Peace Within

Your personal history includes all the words that people, including yourself, have uttered to describe the kind of person you are. Words that cause pain linger on. If you believe there is something fundamentally wrong with you, somewhere along the way, things undoubtedly were said that cut you to the bone. Such words wound because we are sensitive beings, vulnerable to one another. All of us, young and old, yearn to be recognized as precious. Unfortunately, if loving affirmation was in short supply, you may believe that you do not deserve to be treated with love and respect and that you have little to contribute to others. These beliefs are false. You must see through the illusion that you are irreversibly flawed. Here is the bottom line. Any narrative about who you are as a person that causes anxiety is simply not true. When you hear such a story going through your mind, stop what you are doing, breathe deeply, and whisper a calming chant in the same way a mother sings to a baby. Continue until you feel comforted, calm, and aware of feeling quiet deep in your heart.

For this practice, sit meditatively. Lovingly chant, "Shanti, shanti, shanti, Om" or "Peace, peace, peace, amen." Conclude by affirming, "I feel peaceful deep within."

Today I feel peace in my heart.

Who I Am

What you do, say, and experience changes over time. However, the opinions you have about yourself can last for years, and strongly entrenched beliefs about not being lovable enough or smart enough or courageous enough cause great emotional pain. When such viewpoints grow deep roots in your mind, they become part of the core story about who you think you are. In reality, they do not accurately describe who you are. Just because opinions stick around, that does not mean they are the truth. According to the great yogi Ramana Maharishi (Osborne 1972), one of the most revealing yoga practices is answering the question "Who am I?" until you run out of responses and your false self is exposed. Generally, your initial answers include your name, circumstances, roles and responsibilities, prevailing moods, talents, and opinions. Continue on, saying all you can say, until your only remaining answer is "I am," followed by silence. In the silence you meet yourself—alive, aware, and real, and not confined to a set of opinions. You have entered the domain of the true self, where deep inner peace resides.

For this journaling practice, respond to the question "Who am I?" until you exhaust all answers other than "I am." Then sit meditatively, silently, experiencing who you are beneath your opinions. Conclude by affirming, "I am."

Today I experience who I truly am.

I Am Not My Thoughts

When the inner critic attacks, it is easy to forget that you are a spiritual being having a human experience. Thoughts that belittle bring on emotional pain, which can cause you to feel miserable and make you temporarily believe you are a miserable person. In the midst of pain, it is easy to forget that you are also the observer of thoughts and experiences. The Sanskrit words *aham saksih* translate as "I am the eternal witness"; they represent the innermost you that lives on. Everything else, including experiences, thoughts, and the cells of your body, is transitory. You live in your body, but your ever-changing body is not who you are. You live through situations, but they come and go and are not who you are. You have thoughts, but the thousands of thoughts that pass through your mind are not who you are. Remaining always, as you and with you, is the eternal, unalterable witness. When you hear critical thoughts or are hard on yourself, stop, take several deep breaths, then slowly and repeatedly whisper, "I am the witness." This quiets your mind, calms your nerves, and reminds you that you are not your thoughts.

For this practice, sit meditatively. Whisper or chant over and over, "Aham saksih" or "I am the witness." Conclude by affirming, "I witness."

Today I realize that I am not my thoughts.

Who I Am Not

You are profoundly influenced by those close to you; thus you are inevitably wounded when loved ones degrade you. Their words matter to you and can penetrate all the way into the core story of who you think you are. When someone important to you repeatedly says that you are "no good," eventually you begin to believe that you are "no good." Words can have powerful effects whether they are the opinion of others or your own thoughts. No matter what others say, you cannot be reduced to words or stories, yours or anyone else's. You are not a pile of words. You are a sacred human being.

A famous Sanskrit mantra, *Neti, neti,* translates as "Not this, not this." A form of self-inquiry, it points to the truth of who you are by refuting what you are not. This mantra is a powerful shield because when you say, "Neti, neti," in essence you are saying, "These words do not describe me." So when you or someone else says something unkind about you, silently whisper, "Not this, not this." It is freeing to know what you are not, and you certainly are not trash.

For this practice, sit meditatively. Silently recite this mantra for several minutes. Conclude by affirming, "I am a sacred being."

Today I recognize who I am.

My Heart Knows

A child needs to light up her parent's eyes. That is how she knows she is precious. When she does not see that sparkle, sooner or later she may believe she is one of the undesirables. Likewise, an adult can be brainwashed into believing that he is unworthy or that she deserves to be abused. Maltreatment can lead you to believe that you are not among the chosen and may cause you to doubt the existence of the divine. This kind of suffering makes you feel terribly alone and abandoned. Only divine love heals this suffering. Its warmth penetrates the quiet depths of your heart, where it moves hurt out and lets compassion in. This profound love is always available to you. Your heart knows how precious you are because in your heart you feel the loving presence of the divine as an aspect of yourself. Swami Durgananda (2002) teaches that heart meditation is a profound way to enter into your sacred heart.

For this practice, sit meditatively. Breathe in and out from the bottom of your heart. Concentrate on your heart. Enter it, going deep within. Feel its tender warmth and linger there. Conclude by affirming, "I feel the presence of divine love."

Today I feel love in my heart.

The Light Within

You have a transcendent core that remains even when it has been covered over with thick layers of untruths. You may not be aware of your inner radiance, but it is there. Your task is to find it, to dig below the surface, to go beneath shame, doubt, and pain. Under the muck, your inner essence is pure gold.

Finding lost art and uncovering your inner radiance both feel miraculous. Yet both usually require personal effort. Centuries ago monks covered a golden Buddha statue in Thailand with eight to twelve inches of clay to protect it from being looted by the invading Burmese army. The army killed all the monks, and the beautiful Buddha was lost to history. Then, in 1957, the statue was dropped while being moved. A monk inspecting the damaged statue shone a flashlight into a crack and saw brilliant gold. Monks then chiseled off the clay, discovered the Buddha, and bowed in awe. The Sanskrit mantra *So 'ham* means "I am that" (referring to transcendent self). Like hastening a miracle waiting to happen, reciting this mantra shines a flashlight into the radiance within.

For this practice, sit meditatively. Silently chant or whisper "sooooo" while inhaling and "hummmm" while exhaling. Repeat over and over and over again. Conclude by affirming, "I bow to the light within."

Today I honor the radiance within.

Choosing My Higher Self

You have free will and can choose your primary identity. Your false self, so filled with expectations, seeks happiness in fulfilling instinctual needs for security, esteem, and control (Keating 2009). Sadly, this is the only identity some people know. The true you—your higher self, who is not masked by expectations—recognizes life as sacred, experiences oneness with all life, and wants only to serve the divine. When you choose to identify with this innermost self, your choice helps you hold the misunderstandings of your false self in love, which, over time, dissipates the emotional force field encircling that false self. So when the pain of your false self overtakes you, which you experience as fear, despair, or the loneliness of inferiority or superiority, utilize your free will. First stop, pause, and take a few deep breaths. Then choose to identify with your higher self. One way to do so is by chanting the mantra *Om, namah shivaya*, translated as "I bow to the inner true self, the consciousness that dwells in all." Repeat over and over and over again, until you feel soothed and calm inside.

For this practice, sit meditatively. Chant or sing "Om, namah shivaya" for several minutes. Then sit quietly, absorbed in peaceful inner quiet. Conclude by affirming, "I hold my pain in love and let truth shine through."

Today I choose to be more than my false self.

My Body Is My Home

You reveal your opinions about your appearance with the comments you make standing in front of a mirror. Nonetheless, you cannot be reduced to your body, much less to how it looks. Our culture, preoccupied with image, links identity to physical appearance, especially for women. This emphasis causes eating disorders, low self-esteem, fear of aging, and more. You are close to your body. You feel it, see it, touch it, and your human life depends upon it, yet you are not defined by your body. You have many bodies during your time on earth. The body's tissues are under constant renewal, and your skeletal cells are replaced every seven years.

You live inside your body. It is important to honor and respect your body, to treat it like the holy place it is. However, after weighing your worth on the scales of society-sanctioned attractiveness, back away. Chant the Sanskrit mantra *Sri Ram, Jai Ram, Jai Jai Ram,* or in English, "May the Lord of light and virtue that dwells in my heart be victorious over all," so you remember who you are and can soothe the pain of identifying with your body.

For this practice, sit meditatively. Chant "Sri Ram, Jai Ram, Jai Jai Ram" many, many times. Then sit and enjoy silence. Conclude by affirming, "I love my body; it is my home."

Today I honor my body as home.

My Peaceful Core

Peace is not something outside yourself that you earn and then add on. It is inside you, and it becomes available when you let go of trying to make yourself into a peaceful person. It's what remains after you let go of your belief that peace is available in the future when you accomplish certain goals. Your false identity deeply yearns for peace and does not know that true serenity arises from within. It searches for peace by accumulating extra stuff in your home and closet and completing to-do lists. These efforts are as effective as trying to make a diamond sparkle by burying it in manure. Peace arises naturally when you release your efforts to earn peace. Your innermost self is already peaceful. Nothing is missing; nothing needs to be added on. Therefore, the way to peace is emptying out, subtracting what is not needed. Peace is an inner diamond waiting to be discovered. Spiritual practices like meditation, prayer, chanting, and devotional singing strip away what is unnecessary, uncovering your peaceful core.

For this practice, sit meditatively. After a few minutes, recite a favorite prayer, repeat a chant, or sing a devotional song that connects you to that quiet state deep within. Then sit for ten or more minutes, absorbed in stillness. Conclude by affirming, "I feel peaceful."

Today I uncover my peaceful core.

chapter 2

Root Chakra

Body and mind live together in unity, each reflecting the state of the other. It follows, then, that when you feel safe in your body, you feel safe in your mind. Feeling safe in your body pertains to the root chakra, which is about your most basic survival needs and your sense of belonging to family, community, and the world around you. The Sanskrit name for this chakra is *Muladhara*, which translates as "root support" or "foundation." Located at the base of your spine, it is the foundational chakra for your energetic system. Intertwined with your connection to your physical body, your family, and even the earth that sustains life, Muladhara is the energy that anchors you to your flesh and bones and enables you to live out your life on earth as a spirit in human form.

The element associated with the root chakra is earth, which shelters and provides for human life. Its energy is strength, the kind that allows you to stand on your own feet and to feel connection. It is also your survival center, your primal drive to protect and be safe. Basically, this energy enables you to tend to your basic needs and those of your loved ones. As such, it is the most instinctual of the chakras. Accordingly, it is the energy that activates your fight-flight-freeze response when danger is sensed.

Energy in the root chakra can become blocked as a result of trauma—most notably, mistreatment in early life, including physical neglect and abuse, parental loss through divorce or death, and survival threats, but also traumas that threaten your safety during adult life. Blockage in this area can cause chronic fear, anxiety, and worry. Additionally, when its energetic flow is blocked, you may feel as though you do not belong and may struggle with fatigue, money, jobs, and relationships. When your root chakra is strong, clear, and balanced, you feel secure and stable and enjoy a sense of family and community.

Life energy can take various forms. You do not have to be dominated by the energy of fear, becoming lost in the sense of isolation that arises with fear. You can lessen the impact of fear by tapping into tremendous reserves of stability, fortitude, and triumph, which are the energy of the earth. The energy of Muladhara allows you to be courageous and resourceful during challenging times, as it connects you to the enduring energy of the earth, the grit of family ancestors, and the immense spiritual muscle of great beings and teachers who have gone before.

The meditations in this chapter open, balance, and stimulate your root chakra. Try them all, then select a few that you find most appealing and practice them faithfully for a month or more. Above all, remember that you are here, you are supported, you have access to tremendous strength, and your life matters.

Accessing Inner Strength

When you are motivated by unconscious fear, you may attempt to control loved ones. It's as if asserting dominance over others makes you feel safer. However, these efforts deplete the energy you need to develop your own strengths. Such behavior indicates imbalance in your root chakra. You can lessen your emotional need to fix or otherwise be in charge of others by stimulating your root chakra, which increases your sense of inner security. One way to do so is a yantra meditation, where you gaze at the image of a large land mammal who is strong and protective of its young—the elephant. The sacred elephant often appears in images of the root chakra. Considered royal, the elephant tends to live in a family group, ensuring survival and longevity, and is known for prowess in war. Accordingly, accessing elephant energy helps you feel as protected as a growing elephant calf surrounded by its herd while it develops and matures.

To practice, sit meditatively. Place an image of an elephant at eye level and gaze at it steadily and calmly. Alternatively, visualize an elephant in your mind's eye. Feel its sturdiness, steadiness, and loyalty. Then sit quietly and feel the presence of regal elephant energy. To conclude, affirm, "I feel protected by the strength of the sacred elephant."

Today I feel safe and strong.

Centering in My Body

Unresolved fear, the emotion most associated with insufficiency in the root chakra, is expressed through your nervous system. In attempting to ensure your safety, your nervous system may become hypervigilant, causing you to frequently scan the environment for signs of danger and startle at even slight rustling. As a result, you tend to notice more what is going on around you and less what is going on inside you, such as the sensations associated with the touch of your feet on the floor. Paradoxically, this causes you to feel ungrounded and therefore less safe. The following practice entails focusing attention in your lower body, at the base of your spine. This calms your nerves and helps you be aware of being in your body. As a result, you feel more grounded and at ease.

To practice, sit meditatively. If comfortable, sit with one heel placed beneath your pelvic floor at the perineum. Alternatively, place a folded washcloth under your pelvic floor so that you experience slight pressure in that area, or simply focus on your hips or sit bones. Modify your posture as needed for comfort. Center your attention on the pressure point and take ten comfortable breaths. Then sit quietly and enjoy feeling grounded. Conclude by affirming, "I feel calm and stable and in my body."

Today I feel centered in my body.

Feeling Rooted

When you have not felt safe for a long time, you may become overly concerned with security. Then fear becomes a central feature in your personality that lives on after the old turmoil is gone. Unintentionally, you act as though life were threatening, when, in reality, your circumstances are now stable and you have greater capacity to take care of yourself. This kind of embedded fear can show up as workaholism, stubbornness, and difficulty with change, or other tendencies that restrict your ability to grow and expand. Although there usually are real challenges in life, there is enough support available to help you navigate your way through them in positive ways. Opening the root chakra allows you to access support from within and without. A visualization that opens the root center is imagining that you are a sturdy tree supported by deep roots.

To practice, sit meditatively outdoors or sit and look at a tree through a window. Envision the roots receiving moisture and sustenance from far below. Contemplate how even when a strong wind shakes the branches, the roots are secure and undisturbed. Now imagine yourself going deep within, down through your trunk into your roots, where you are protected, nourished, and safe. After several minutes, release the contemplation. Sit quietly and enjoy your own deep roots. Conclude by affirming, "I feel supported and secure."

Today I access my own deep roots.

Belonging Here

Feeling lonely and thinking you are all alone is as painful as feeling different and thinking you don't fit in. These distressing states can be fleeting; however, often they are long lasting and reflect previous relationship trauma. Whether or not you know it, you do belong; you are never alone. Grounding practices, such as walking meditation, open Muladhara energy and help you realize that, just like hills and trees, you belong here. These insights help you feel okay and enable you to reach out to others.

To practice walking meditation, select a pleasant, safe path to walk, such as the path to your mailbox or the backyard. Alternatively, select a hallway or walk from room to room. Go barefoot, if doing so is comfortable, to enhance the sensations on the soles of your feet. Walk deliberately and feel your feet contacting the earth or floor. Take two to three steps as you slowly inhale and two to three steps as you slowly exhale. Continue walking for ten or more minutes, then sit comfortably for a few minutes and contemplate the truth: that you are being sustained by life and you are never alone. The earth holds you, gravity presses on you, and air surrounds you. Conclude by affirming, "I am here and I belong."

Today I walk the path of belonging.

My Right to Exist

Oppression and violence are massive forces that cause untold suffering. Recent, past, or even inherited trauma, such as war, social injustice, or extreme poverty, can make you doubt your right to be and suck out your life energy. If you lived through such circumstances and are reading this, you survived. You are here. Your right to exist is evidenced by the fact that you still have life. In reality, your life energy does not have to be dictated by the past, no matter what happened. Gently, gradually, and with persistence, you can reclaim your sense of human dignity, which in the end comes from within. The following meditation, on an element of the earth, activates Muladhara energy, which helps you appreciate that you do have a right to be here.

To practice, sit meditatively. Hold something that comes from the earth—perhaps a hand-sized polished stone or rough rock. Feel the object's density, its stillness, and its stable, enduring energy, along with its capacity to withstand changing seasons and periodic storms. Sit quietly and let yourself be nurtured by quiet, steadfast earth energy. Breathe in its strength. Recognize that the energy of the earth is in you. Place the object on a table or in your pocket so that you have a reminder throughout the day. Conclude by affirming, "My strength comes from powerful energy within."

Today I reclaim my right to be here.

Standing My Ground

Weak stick-to-itiveness often reflects previous struggle and disadvantage in your life or in the lives of your extended family. If an energy of overwhelming odds, tough blows, and "not much is possible" circles around you, know that you are not destined to perpetuate patterns of resignation. You can learn to keep your feet on the ground and move toward a better future. Just because being discouraged is familiar does not mean that the energy of steadfastness is not available. Perseverance is inches away, as close as the earth. One way to draw upon earth energy is practicing mountain pose, the most basic standing pose in yoga, where you stand tall with both feet planted on the earth or the floor. Practice this pose faithfully to receive regular doses of standing your ground.

To practice, stand barefoot, with your feet hip width apart, on the earth or floor. Lengthen your spine and let your shoulders, torso, and neck relax. Rest your arms at your sides, palms facing forward. Press your feet onto the earth beneath you. Lift your toes, spread them out, and place them back on the earth or floor. Imagine roots extending down from your feet into the soil. Stand as firm as a mountain and breathe fully. Conclude by affirming, "I am steadfast, and I can stand my ground."

Today I am standing on solid ground.

Claiming My Boundaries

No matter what has or has not happened to you, you are here. You still have a physical body. Even though we are all connected, you have your life to take care of, which is easier when you feel solidly at home in your body. When you sense where you end and others begin, you are more able to stand up for yourself. Then you are able to say "mine" and mean it. This helps reduce the fear that goes with not having personal boundaries and not feeling the strength to set limits. If you are not aware of your physical boundaries, you leave space for others to intrude and take advantage of you. Then you may feel depleted or controlled by others or experience difficulty ending unhealthy relationships. When this happens, you have little energy left to tend to yourself and what is important to you. Practicing *mula bandha*, or the root lock, makes you aware of your physical boundaries. It is performed by contracting the perineum muscles, located between the anus and genitals.

To practice, sit meditatively in a quiet room. Breathe in and pause. Pull your pelvic floor muscles up and inward, hold for a moment, then relax the muscles while exhaling. Practice for a few minutes. Then softly chant several rounds of "Mine, mine, mine." Conclude by affirming, "I have boundaries."

Today I claim my boundaries.

Receiving Support

You know fear; it is your body's instinctual response to perceived danger. As a child, you turned to trusted adults, if they were available, for protection when your well-being was threatened. Even as an adult, with all your capacities, it is much easier to face fear and fight important battles when you feel supported. Muladhara energy helps you be brave and resourceful, and even provides the will to live during challenging times. You do not ever have to go it alone. Help is available whenever you need it, including times when you are overwhelmed by daunting circumstances, such as when you need to defend loved ones, navigate your way through difficult transitions, or change a destructive habit. Summon the strength of Muladhara by calling upon your primary spiritual ancestors, whatever your religious background. One example is the mighty force of

Durga, the Indian warrior goddess of strength and protection. Alternatively, if you do not consider yourself spiritual, call upon a great person whose wisdom and power deeply touch you.

To practice, sit quietly with your pen and journal. Describe your difficulty and the type of support you need. Next, visualize yourself sitting in front of your spiritual ancestor. Reverently bow before him or her. Breathe in the strength you need and breathe out fear and negativity. Conclude by affirming, "I welcome support."

Today I call upon my spiritual ancestor for support.

Feeling Grounded

Body and mind have a profound impact on each other. One way their interconnectedness manifests is the disturbed relationship with eating that sometimes comes in the aftermath of emotional mistreatment and neglect. When you are hurt by the ones you love and they are not available to comfort you, you may turn to food as a substitute for support. This sets in motion a painful cycle between body and mind. Unhealthy eating leads to self-loathing, which in turn creates emotional distress and the need for soothing. Before long this pattern may weaken your ability to make and stick with healthy food choices. Strengthening your root chakra energy by consuming grounding foods—root vegetables like potatoes, carrots, and beets, as well as earthy foods like nuts, beans, and legumes—helps cultivate a healthy body-mind food cycle. However, eating disturbances become entrenched. Being able to make wise food choices involves taking time daily to stabilize your mind and mood. *Juana mudra*, a hand gesture, will connect you to the earth and steady your mind.

To practice, sit meditatively. Feel your hips on the chair and your feet on the floor. Rest your hands on your knees. Join the tips of your thumb and index finger. Point your fingers down toward the earth. Sit quietly for several minutes. Conclude by affirming, "I feel grounded."

Today I stabilize my body and mind.

chapter 3

Sacral Chakra

Make contact with your internal sanctuary, where you feel safe and quiet and your mind can rest more easily. In truth, having access to stillness within makes it much easier to have a peaceful mind in the midst of life's ups and downs. When you know that you can take shelter deep inside, no matter what is happening around you, you are more able to make peace with the way life is and creatively engage with it.

Your inner home is in your sacral chakra. The Sanskrit name for this chakra, *Svadhisthana,* is translated as "one's own sweet place" or "the sacred dwelling place of the self." The sacral chakra is located in the kidney and genital region, which is very close to the first chakra. It is also the base of your creativity, pleasure, morality, and sexuality.

The element associated with the sacral chakra is water. Water yields, goes with the current, and influences everything it flows over. Water represents your great capacity to be fluid, to meet life where it is, and to use your involvement to enhance life around you.

Being able to rest within yourself as quietly as a child napping in her mother's arms is essential to your well-being. Knowing that you can take shelter during inevitable times of upheaval helps you accept the passing seasons of life. Knowing that you can sit alone and quiet your soul helps keep you calm, making it possible for you to enjoy simple sensory pleasures without chasing after them for comfort or meaning. This reduces cravings and addiction to busyness, food, sex, alcohol, adrenaline, and other substances. When you need to soothe your emotional distress, you can take refuge within rather than numbing yourself with carbohydrates or intoxicants. And when you feel bored or disengaged, you can rest in inner stillness and let yourself be recharged and filled again with vitality.

This chakra is sensitive to emotional mistreatment, especially that which occurs in family life. It is particularly sensitive to traumas during your formative years but can also be unbalanced by adult abuse. Suffering sexual abuse or emotional neglect and having your innermost feelings denied can wound, no matter your age. So can religious guilt and indoctrination in severe, punitive moral codes. The lingering effects of such abuse may include feeling guilty about experiencing natural pleasures, such as sexual intimacy in a loving and committed relationship. Mistreatment can drown your enthusiasm for life and wash away your ability to enjoy simple pleasures. It can also cause you to ride the waves of strong emotions or turn sensory gratification into addiction.

Your sacral chakra allows you to feel inner stillness and the movement of life, as well as the dynamic relationship between the two. When it is balanced, you experience contentment from within. Then, even when life is challenging, you remain aware of internal quiet deep in your body. It's a powerful experience to be profoundly touched by life without suffering charged emotional reactivity. It is also wonderful to be able to tap into your talents and, in your unique way, be creative in your life.

Coming Home

In some Eastern traditions, the sacral chakra is named *Hara*. This is the center of your being, through which you make contact with deep stillness and wisdom. It is your energetic home, and it serves to protect and create life and fulfill your life's purpose. Unintentionally, when you are not aware of the still place within, you may seek sensory gratification, through food, alcohol, sex, or drugs, to feel alive or to experience meaning. In contrast, if you seek fulfillment in silence, you become a yogi—one who goes with the flow of life, enjoys pleasure without chasing after it, and rests in the peace of stillness. The physical holy place of the sacral center is situated in your pelvic bowl, in front of your sacrum. The first practice is locating this center.

To practice, sit meditatively. Using your index finger, move down the lower part of your abdomen, beneath your navel, until you come to your pubic bone, the bony portion at the front of the pelvis. Press firmly on the upper part of this bone for about a minute. Visualize the pelvic bowl on the inner side of your public bone. Then remove your finger and, using your inner awareness, concentrate on the location of the sacral chakra. To conclude, affirm, "I come home to the still place within."

Today I feel peaceful and still within.

Moving with Life

Everything gives way. People change; events come and go. However, when your sacral chakra is not open or balanced, you may find yourself holding onto things the way they were. If this describes you, you may feel as though you can't change. You may have little initiative to take the steps that deep inside you know are necessary. Such clinging keeps you stuck, resisting the ways life has moved on. Struggle against the currents of change and you hold onto the past, to the life that is no more. One way to restore your ability to embrace the unending movement of life is to meditate on the image of a luminous orange circle, one symbol for this chakra.

To practice, sit meditatively. Envision a beautiful orange sphere in your mind's eye or gaze at a picture of the harvest moon. Move your eyes around its perimeter, noticing that it has no beginning and no end. Contemplate its wholeness as well as its ability to shapeshift and pass through space. Absorb the brilliant orange color, which symbolizes vitality and creativity, energies that help you find your way. After a few minutes, release the image and sit quietly. See yourself as curious about life and willing to move with the currents of change. Conclude by affirming, "I am finding my way."

Today I move with the ongoing flow of life.

Washing Away Guilt

Deep inside, your inner home of stillness is undisturbed. However, your thoughts and emotions can feel impure because, like water, they may carry impurities. Fortunately, the existence of mud does not change the basic nature of water, nor does it contaminate your inner essence. Nonetheless, thoughts about being unclean and feelings of guilt are strong energies that may prevent you from experiencing pleasure as a natural aspect of being human. A strict moral upbringing or being scolded as an adult for enjoying music, food, dance, or sex can cause you to feel guilty about experiencing these simple pleasures. You do not have to remain shut off from bodily pleasure. Water, the element associated with the sacral chakra, is flowing, flexible, and adaptive. Soft and yielding, water purifies what it touches. Bathing removes dirt from your skin; in a similar manner, meditating on the cleansing nature of water can wash away guilt.

To practice, sit meditatively. Envision sitting on a sandy shore with warm ocean waves that gently lap over your ankles and legs, then recede back into the ocean. Imagine that each wave draws guilt into it and then carries it away. After a few minutes, release the image and sit quietly, feeling emotionally cleansed. Conclude by affirming, "It is my nature to enjoy simple pleasures."

Today I wash away guilt.

Releasing Negativity

When you are mired in recurring negative thoughts, such as "It won't work" or "I don't have enough energy," you may give up on your dreams and not do the things that truly matter to you. Then you end up feeling discouraged or frustrated and become stuck in a rut. Negativity is a big energy drainer whether it is created by mutual complaining with others or by yourself, in your own mind. Either way, if you surround yourself with negativity, your inner desires may be flushed away. Walk away from negative conversations, and use the following meditation to disengage from negativity and balance your sacral chakra.

To practice, sit meditatively. Bring to mind a couple of negative thoughts that bother you. In your mind's eye, see yourself sitting on the bank of a river. Place each negative thought on a leaf going downstream and watch the current carry it away. Sit quietly for several minutes; if another negative thought comes to mind, place it on a leaf and watch it float away. Notice the growing distance between you and those thoughts. Unattached to negative thoughts, you are free to move. Enjoy this peaceful feeling. Conclude by smiling softly and affirming, "I am moving on."

Today I let go of my negative thoughts.

Looking for Happiness

Yearning to be happy is a deep desire. However, seeking happiness through sensory pleasure is misguided. Lasting happiness does not come from grasping for food, sex, alcohol, drugs, or the comforts of money. Sensory desires can only be temporarily gratified. When happiness is sought through their fulfillment, you need to have more and more. The drive to consume can take over, and you lose sight of contentment from deep within. This results in indulgences and addictions, indicating imbalance in the sacral chakra. Balancing your sacral chakra helps you become aware of deep inner stillness, far beneath restless cravings, which is the true source of happiness. The still, radiant, white crescent moon, reflecting only a sliver of the moon, is a symbol of the sacral chakra. The moon governs the tides and flow of water, reflects the light of the sun, and represents the movement and vitality necessary for life. Meditating on the crescent moon can help you experience inner stillness and be satisfied with simple pleasures.

To practice, sit meditatively. With eyes closed, envision the shining crescent moon, its gravitational pull and unending orbit. Then move your attention deep inside. From inner stillness, sense the mysterious unending movement of life. Conclude by affirming, "Simple pleasures satisfy me."

Today I feel happy deep inside.

Tasting Life's Sweetness

At times the experience of living is as flavorful as the taste of sun-ripened fruit. Although sorrow and difficulty are a part of the mix, life can be seasoned with laughter, friendships, celebrations, and sweet surprises. It is in these things that you sense life's loveliness; otherwise life can lose its richness and texture and seem flat. When the sacral chakra's energy is blocked, you can feel numb and socially cut off, and you miss out on the pleasing aspects of life. When you lack enthusiasm, little seems interesting, and depression can ensue. Taste is the sense associated with your sacral chakra. Foods that balance this chakra include orange foods like mango, mandarin oranges, carrots, and yams, as well as other tropical fruits, seeds, nuts, fish, sweet honey, and even chocolate. A food-tasting meditation is useful for opening the sacral chakra.

To practice, select a few of the foods listed. Arrange the food on a colorful plate or napkin and place on a table in front of you. Sit quietly for a minute or so. Next, take a bite of the food. Eat slowly and really savor it. Notice texture, flavor, temperature, and moisture in your mouth. Swallow and take another bite. Continue until finished. Contemplate the pleasing tastes of food and of life. Conclude by affirming, "I embrace life's loveliness."

Today I celebrate life's sweetness.

Daring to Dream

You have tremendous capacity to create loving homes, meaningful careers, refreshing vacations, and more. Sometimes when you dare to dream, inner guidance reveals ways to develop your talents and fulfill your life's purpose. However, when the sacral chakra is out of balance, your capacity to dream, be hopeful, and even make mistakes is dampened. Then, when you feel like you are at a dead end, home, work, play, and inner life can become boring and mechanical. You fall out of sync with the creative movement of life. One way to balance your sacral chakra is with a simple yoga practice, where you flow from one pose to another.

To practice, wear clothing that allows movement. Sit in a straight-back chair with your feet on the floor and your knees at least hip width apart. Breathing in, lift your arms overhead and reach your chest toward the sky. Breathing out, bring your arms down by your heart, and then slide them down your legs as you lean over and rest your chest by your legs in a forward fold. Repeat this gentle flowing movement five or more times. Move slowly and easily. To finish, stay in the forward fold for a few breaths. Return to a comfortable seated position and sit quietly for several minutes. Conclude by affirming, "I can dream little and I can dream big."

Today I let myself dream.

Learning to Be Still

You can transform your life. However, making beneficial changes requires both stillness and creative impulse. Without stillness, change can be a knee-jerk reaction to fear, restlessness, or guilt that may not move you in a desirable direction. When change arises out of inner stillness, it is worthwhile for you and for others. True creativity requires entering into not knowing, letting go of certainty, and learning to tolerate ambiguity and paradox, which are all easier to do when you can sit quietly with yourself and wait. Giving yourself time and not rushing helps you hear the wisdom that arises out of stillness. When your sacral chakra is imbalanced, your ability to be still is diminished. One way to balance your sacral chakra is by meditating on an image of a white water lily. Not adapted to fast-moving water, this hardy plant flourishes in still ponds of freshwater. Its delicate petals open with the rising sun and close with the setting sun. The beautiful lily symbolizes truth, spirituality, pleasure, and rebirth.

To practice, sit meditatively. Gaze at a picture of a white water lily or see one in your mind's eye. Envision its roots at home in the dark, still bottom of the pond and its flowers nestled amid floating leaves. Then close your eyes and sit quietly. Conclude by affirming, "I sit quietly."

Today I am learning to be still.

Taking Refuge

Circumstances can change dramatically, unexpectedly, and rapidly, causing you to feel overwhelmed. When this occurs, you can benefit by taking refuge from the storm of strong emotions so you can respond wisely to events that affect you. Other times you may have turbulent emotions even when life is calm on the outside. Whatever their cause, when strong emotions come flooding in, your sacral chakra may be or become imbalanced. To balance the sacral chakra and create internal refuge, sit quietly and practice the water mudra (or hand gesture) called *varun*. In this mudra, your thumb and little finger form a circle, which symbolizes eternal movement as well as containment. Focusing intently on this hand gesture steadies your attention, calms your nerves, and helps you ride waves of emotion without being swallowed up by them.

To practice, sit meditatively. Rest the backs of your hands on your thighs. Join the tips of your little fingers and thumbs, applying enough pressure to feel the pulse between them. Relax your other fingers. Turn your palms face up, representing receptivity to life. Imagine being open to the changing currents of life while simultaneously feeling stillness deep within. Focus intently on your hands and the mudra, then sit quietly for a few minutes. Conclude by affirming, "I steady myself when my emotions run high."

Today I take refuge in stillness.

chapter 4

Solar Plexus Chakra

Having a peaceful mind becomes possible when you feel that you and your life matter. In fact, it is crucial to know that you have value, because then you have the initiative, resolve, and confidence to act on what is important to you. When your solar plexus chakra, which is located between your navel and spine, is balanced, the spark of your unique character is ignited. Your personal capacities and talents begin to shine, and you participate more wholeheartedly in life. The Sanskrit name for this chakra is *Manipuri,* translated as "city of jewels." To appreciate the energy of Manipuri, imagine a treasure chest deep in your belly shimmering with clarity, self-assurance, love of life, plus much more.

The Manipuri chakra supports your ability to listen to your gut instincts, a source of intuitive guidance that, when followed, enhances the quality of life—yours as well as others'. Irrational, emotionally reactive calls to action can disguise themselves as gut instinct. That is why learning discernment—the ability to see and understand your emotional tendencies, which helps you avoid basing important life decisions on them—is so beneficial. The illuminating light of Manipuri helps you see your shame, self-protection, fear, and insecurity so that you do not pass on your pain to others. It also shows you what your deeper desires are so you know what to act on. And it lets you appreciate that everyone has unique value and potential.

Not only does your solar plexus chakra reveal old emotional motivations and show you the steps you need to take; it gives you the self-confidence to take those steps. The animal symbol for Manipuri is a ram, which represents fearlessness, drive, protection, and leadership. This symbol gives a strong sense of the chakra's powerful energy. Knowing what you need to do and having the "ram energy" to do it come together as personal power. Otherwise, you may know what you need to do but lack the ability to act on it. Or you may be able to act but not have inner clarity, which can quickly set your life adrift. The ability to be discerning and the confidence to act wisely go hand in hand.

Like the other energy centers, Manipuri can be affected by trauma. Being shamed, tyrannized, or oppressed can unbalance Manipuri. Those forms of emotional trauma rob you of personal authority, snuff out your love of life, and make you believe the lie that you are unworthy. As a result, you may feel defeated and want to withdraw from life, or you may feel resentful and frustrated and aggressively pursue whatever you want with little regard for others.

The following meditations are designed to fill you with the bright light of discernment, infuse you with vitality, and help you discover your own value in the universe so that your life feels full and rewarding. Along the way, you end up thinking less about yourself and more about how to put your time and energy into what matters.

Honoring My Inner Fire

Having the right amount of heat or "fire" in your belly lights up the best of your character and lets your personality fill with warmth, self-confidence, and the ability to do what matters most to you. If your fire is low, you may feel insecure, find it hard to make decisions, and compare yourself negatively to others. If your fire rages, you may dominate others, have temper flares, and believe you are better than others. By balancing this chakra, you appreciate your unique abilities, yet understand that everyone has talents and that we are all together making our way through life. To balance this chakra, it is helpful to first locate it.

To do so, stand sideways in front of a mirror. Place an index or middle finger on your navel and the same finger of your other hand on your spine, directly behind your navel. Release the finger over your navel while continuing to press on your spine. Next, sit comfortably with your spine upright, pressing on your spine for a minute; then release your finger. Notice the pressure sensation and focus inwardly on the area between your navel and your spine. This is the location of Manipuri. Conclude by affirming, "I want the right amount of fire in my belly."

Today I want to let my best shine through.

Shining a Light in Myself

The color associated with the solar plexus chakra is sunny yellow, and the symbol is an inverted triangle. Imagine a yellow triangle representing light that rises like the golden sun. This chakra governs your thoughts about the kind of person you are, as well as your outlook on life. It is sensitive to the attitudes of your loved ones. If parents or significant people shamed or dominated you, you may view yourself as unworthy and be more of a pessimist than an optimist. These perceptions and attitudes are understandable, given such circumstances, but misguided. In truth, your intrinsic worth cannot be taken away by anyone, not even yourself. You need to see how valuable you are so that your sense of self and your disposition are brought up out of darkness. One way to do so, and to balance this chakra, is with an infusion of yellow light.

For this practice, sit comfortably upright in a sunny location. With eyes closed, picture rays of warm sunlight emanating from within your navel, as if the sun were rising inside you. Envision your body and mind infused with brilliant light. Let brightness burn away negativity and fill you with appreciation for yourself and life. Release the image and bask for a few minutes in the afterglow. Conclude by affirming, "The light of worthiness shines in me."

Today I see that my life matters.

Lighting the Flame of Self-Acceptance

You suffer from perfectionism if you push yourself toward flawlessness, criticize your performance, cringe and try harder, while fearing that your perceived flaws are apparent to others. Perfection is a strong drive, but it is not true personal power because it is based in the need to prove. This pattern indicates imbalance in your solar plexus chakra and is often linked to past experiences of being held to exacting standards, feeling ashamed of your family, or prematurely assuming adult responsibilities. Perfectionism softens in the warmth of understanding, when it is seen as the need to prove worthiness, which can only be experienced, not verified. One way to melt perfection is offering it to the flame of acceptance—a source of incredible personal power—in a fire meditation.

To do this, arrange lit candles on a large nonflammable surface or sit before an open fire. Have pen and paper nearby. Recall a time when you negated a compliment for a good effort or a job well done. Write down this memory. Offer this memory as fuel for self-acceptance, which knows how hard you try. Hold the edge of the paper to the flame, burn through the phrase, and safely drop the paper. Repeat the compliment and finally let it in. Sit for a few minutes, silently watching the fire. Conclude by affirming, "I am enough as I am."

Today I am willing to accept myself as I am.

Accessing Energy

Most people experience low energy and feel discouraged when hard times exhaust them. After all, life can present daunting challenges, and people around you can drag you down emotionally. But when inaction, indecisiveness, and poor follow-through come to define your approach to life, they probably reflect deficient energy in your solar plexus chakra. Here is the bottom line: You are not doomed to a lifetime of passivity. Vast reservoirs of strength and resolve are available to help you go through struggles without giving up on yourself and life. One way to tap into this energy and activate your solar plexus chakra is through the breathing practice called *kapalabhati,* also known as fire breath or shining breath.

To do this, sit up tall and get comfortable. Gently place both hands, one stacked over the other, on your navel area so you feel your abdomen contracting when you breathe out. Take a couple of deep breaths and begin panting like a dog with your mouth open. Then close your mouth and continue practicing this breath through your nose, making a puffing sound as you exhale quickly. Take ten breaths followed by a brief rest. Do two or three more sets. Sit quietly for a few minutes. Conclude by affirming, "I can access the energy I need."

Today I realize that life energy is there for me.

Tempering My Fire

The energy in your belly chakra occasionally flares out of balance and causes irritability. However, when your emotional drive is like a fire constantly on high, it can show up as workaholism, lack of sensitivity to how you affect others, and a tendency to be domineering. You may pursue status and productivity at the price of felt human connectedness. Over time, excess Manipuri energy can push others away and cause you to feel alone, making worldly success truly hollow. When you spend your time and energy to acquire prestige, you are less apt to temper fear-based motivations, such as the desire to be in control and to not need others. You also have less time to truly discover what your heart-based motivations are. This holds you back, because refining your motives empowers you and makes your character shine. Then you touch your own life and the lives of others with generosity, love of life, and reliability.

One way to balance your solar plexus chakra and cultivate heart-based power is by chanting. To practice this, sit meditatively. Focus your attention on your navel. Sing or speak, "Shanti, shanti, shanti, Om" or "Peace, peace, peace, amen" softly for five minutes or more. Then sit quietly and calmly. Conclude by affirming, "I want to refine my motives and mold my character."

Today the power of love moves through me.

Improving My Inner Vision

A child experiences her worthiness when she is treated with love and respect, given freedom to make choices, and protected from harm. If you were degraded or oppressed, you were taught a lie about your place in the universe. The same is true if you were scorned as an adult. The result may be that you view life through the lens of shame, which makes the future look dim. Believing that you are unworthy indicates imbalance in your sacral chakra. Vision, the sense associated with this chakra, pertains to your ability to picture the kind of life that becomes possible when you see yourself as worthy of honorable treatment. One way to purify this chakra is with a breathing practice that will relax you and make envisioning a brighter future easier.

To practice, sit meditatively with eyes closed. Breathe slowly and evenly. As you breathe in, feel your navel expand; as you breathe out, feel your navel contract. After a few rounds, envision breathing in through your navel and out from your navel, gently pulling your abdominal muscles in toward your spine as you exhale. Continue this breathing practice for a minute, then relax. Using inner sight, imagine the life you truly want, including at least one specific change. Conclude by affirming, "I am learning to treat myself and my life with honor."

Today I envision positive changes.

Choosing Love

You become the person you are meant to be by making conscious choices. The most direct path to personal empowerment is making choices every day based on love and trust rather than fear and distrust. Acknowledge old fear-based motives, pat them gently, and then choose to develop your talents and show love. You may feel vulnerable but know that you are okay because you are aligned with what matters rather than with old defensive patterns. This is how your character grows, choice by choice by conscious choice. You will make mistakes. They are part of learning. Simply make new choices as you go. Choosing is the action of Manipuri, and having the inner resolve to follow through on your choices results from balancing this chakra. Spinal-rotation yoga poses help balance this chakra.

For this practice, sit comfortably. Rotate your torso to the left, with your left hand beside your left hip and your right hand on your left knee. Look to the left. Hold the pose, breathe deeply, and see how fear influenced your past. Do the same pose on the right side, breathe deeply, and see how love can influence your future. Repeat on both sides, then sit meditatively. Choose to do something today that expresses love for yourself and life. Conclude by affirming, "I see fear and realize that I can choose love."

Today I practice choosing love over fear.

Choosing What I Consume

Eating wholesome foods keeps your body healthy, and chewing on great thoughts keeps your mind in top shape. Just as you have choice about what you eat, you can select the kinds of thoughts you take in. Your mind is yours to take care of, and it is up to you to nourish it. The quality of your life reflects the quality of your thoughts, and there is no benefit in swallowing toxic thoughts. Reject harmful thoughts the same way you throw away rotten food. Your mental and physical health is dependent on what you consume, and your ability to choose well depends on your solar plexus chakra being balanced. One way to balance this chakra is through conscious food consumption. This cultivates your capacity to make choices that enhance your well-being and the well-being of others. Foods that balance Manipuri include bananas, granola, whole grains, flax, sunflower seeds, cheese, and yogurt.

For this practice, select from the above foods. Give thanks or pray before eating. Smell a spoonful of food, place it in your mouth, and wait a moment. Then eat with your eyes closed, chewing slowly. When finished, sit quietly. Think about great thoughts that generate love, resolve, and optimism. Conclude by affirming, "I choose to eat wholesome foods and thoughts."

Today I practice conscious consumption.

Developing My Potential

Becoming all you can be does not result from seeking fame and fortune. Your potential is about your capacity to give and receive more love. You at your best means doing what matters to your heart, standing up for what you believe in, and appreciating how sacred life truly is. Developing your potential involves transforming your character from one motivated by fear to one motivated by love. Becoming who you are meant to be occurs as you show up in loving ways, moment by moment by moment, and dare to be real and vulnerable and truthful along the path. This kind of change is possible with a little trust, big doses of determination, and small steps day by day. The yoga practice *sankulpa* can help you take transformational steps. It's simple. State what you want to cultivate, then write down one thing you can do each day to develop that quality. And remember, actions motivated by reverence for life let the best of you shine through.

To practice, put a pen and paper nearby. Sit meditatively. Consider what you truly desire—for example, to express love freely. Write your desire on paper. Then write down one thing you can do daily to act on your desire—for example, to sing a favorite love song to yourself or someone else. Post your *sankulpa* where you will see it several times daily. Conclude by affirming, "I will do something that really matters today."

Today I set my intention to grow.

chapter 5

Heart Chakra

You can truly know peace when your heart chakra is open—because peace in your mind is felt in your body when there is love in your heart. Your heart, in the center of the chakra system, links the physical and spiritual realms and marks the place where preoccupations with security and appearance give way to the crucial matters of your soul. It makes sense, then, that the opening of your heart coincides with being on a spiritual quest and yearning to experience deep love for yourself and others. This chakra is so central to peace that those who meditate on the heart are considered foremost among yogis.

Your heart is a great healer. The Sanskrit name for the heart center, *Anahata*, means "unhurt" or "unstruck."

Its name implies that in your heart's core, beneath your human vulnerability and inconsolable pain, deep compassion, wholeness, and indescribable peace reside. Like air—the element associated with this center—spiritual energies of your heart permeate the space around it. Since this chakra is shared by emotions and spirit, this is where you approach painful emotions, rather than leaving them unattended. Here is where you embrace fear and despair with the warmth of compassion, in a tender hug that heals. This chakra comforts pain and gives you courage to follow your heart.

The image representing this chakra is a six-pointed star that consists of an upward-pointing triangle superimposed on a downward-pointing triangle. The upward-pointing triangle represents spiritual consciousness, and the downward-pointing triangle represents the material world, including emotions and desires. In the center of the star is an unwavering eternal flame that symbolizes your individual spirit. Here you begin to understand that you are fundamentally a spiritual being on a journey toward love.

This chakra is affected by emotional trauma, especially the death of loved ones, divorce, abandonment, and other losses that tug at or rip your heart. Trauma reverberates through this chakra, causing imbalances that show up in many forms, including obsession with other people's problems, hopelessness, emotional instability, and withholding of love.

Your heart energy is sensitive, so it is important to surround yourself with people who are kind and who recognize the underlying spiritual nature of life. It is equally important to fill your mind with loving thoughts, because the kind of thoughts you have and how often you have them profoundly affect your heart. One symbol of this chakra is an antelope, an animal known for being alert. This symbol encourages you to notice, then move away from thoughts that are pessimistic and bitter, those that cause fear, and to embrace ideas, from within as well as from others, that fill you with optimism and hope.

When the heart chakra is awakened, you experience emotional balance. You talk more lovingly and wisely to yourself and others. Worldly things become less important. You understand that pain and suffering exist, yet you also experience peace and compassion deep within. You feel attuned to the sacred, and your mind becomes more calm and peaceful.

Receiving My Heart

Handing fear, guilt, and sorrow over to the compassion that lives in your heart is profoundly healing. Doing so prompts infinite kindness, letting you know you are never alone and are always loved. The magnitude of your heart chakra's energy not only transforms suffering; it does a whole lot more. It fills you with joy and inspires arts such as music, painting, sculpture, and dance. Your heart chakra, which is located close to your biological heart, exists beyond the physical dimension. In this meditation, you locate and acknowledge your heart of hearts, the symbolic space deep within your chest where divine love resides.

To do this, you will need a washcloth. Sit upright in a chair with firm back support. Place a rolled-up washcloth between the back of your chair and your spine, directly behind your heart. Place one or two fingers on the center of your chest, in front of your heart. Press your fingers into your chest and lean your back into the washcloth for a minute or so. Close your eyes and feel the sensations deep within the spinal column behind your chest. Sit meditatively for several minutes. Then conclude by affirming, "I feel and receive my heart."

Today I greet my inner heart.

Opening My Heart

Unbearable emotions such as intense rejection, fear, and grief can close the door to your heart, which makes you feel even more empty and cold. Then, hopefully, the day comes when you can't take any more. Inconsolable and bereft, you fall to your knees and sob, not knowing what else to do. When you do, your tears open your heart so that compassion can hold anguish in its arms. Fortunately, you do not have to wait for intense pain to open the door of your heart. A symbol of this chakra is an emerald lotus with twelve petals. The color emerald represents healing, love, and hope, and the petals typify the divine energies of this chakra. The following practice will help you gently move into your heart so your suffering can be held with kindness and understanding.

To practice, sit meditatively in a quiet room. Close your eyes, and breathe slowly and deeply. Place one or both hands on your heart and bow. Breathe into and out from the bottom of your heart. Imagine a beautiful emerald lotus in your heart filled with petals of peace, understanding, empathy, purity, kindness, forgiveness, contentment, and joy. Sit quietly and appreciate your heart. Conclude by affirming, "I need my loving heart."

Today I open the door to my heart.

Connecting to Divine Love

Most people feel bitter at one time or another. Long-lasting bitterness causes you to withdraw socially, which leads to the heartache of loneliness. Then you have the sad thought that you don't belong. Isolation and bitterness feed on each other, which in turn makes it difficult to let others in. Yet everyone needs to be loved. Paradoxically, only a loving relationship can melt bitterness. There is a love deep inside that is close, personalized for you, and always available. This love, the love of God, is as close as prayer. One way to connect to divine love is by continuously repeating your chosen name for the divine. This practice of mantra recitation, or *ajapa*, is also called prayer of the heart. Repeating this holy name draws you into its love. Simply stated, when you whisper the name of the divine as a prayer, you begin to feel divine love.

Frequent repetition imprints the word in your mind. Then it spontaneously repeats itself and keeps your heart warm.

To practice mantra recitation, sit meditatively in a quiet room. Become aware of your breathing. Silently recite the word that for you most represents divinity. Repeat it many times, then sit quietly and feel the stirring in your inner heart. Conclude by affirming, "I want to be loved."

Today I repeat the prayer of my heart.

Entering into My Heart

Not knowing that the acceptance and love you yearn for is available within is tragic. You need other people and are profoundly affected by others, yet you need the care that comes from your inner heart as much, if not more. Here is some insight that may move you toward increased self-love. Your thinking mind—not your heart—judges, compares, and berates. Your heart accepts, understands, and forgives, and it can do so wordlessly, through its energy. When you do not feel self-love, it is because you are tormented by pain-producing thoughts, not because there is something wrong with your heart. Fortunately, resting your attention on your heart causes its energy to swell and disturbing thoughts to subside. The following meditation will help you enter into your heart space.

Sit meditatively in a quiet location and close your eyes. Breathe comfortably into and out from your heart. Place one or both hands over your heart. Press gently and feel your heart from the outside. Now put your attention inside your heart. Imagine its warmth radiating and its size expanding. Remain in this state of focused attention. When you are ready, open your eyes. Sit quietly for a few more minutes, basking in your heart energy. Conclude by affirming, "I feel love from within my heart."

Today I rest in my heart.

Offering Compassion

Everybody needs compassion, including you. Extend compassion to yourself, and your heart will melt anxiety and despair the way the springtime sun melts snow. You don't even have to feel deserving of compassion for the wise part of you to extend kind wishes to the part of you that suffers. Simply bring to mind some difficulty you are having. Then think of someone else who has similar problems and send sincere wishes of healing to her or him. This gets the "compassion juices going" and helps you realize that everyone has difficulties and deserves compassion. It is then easier to offer compassion to yourself. All you do is send wishes of happiness and health to yourself. Your heart responds and does the rest.

To practice, sit in a meditative posture and recite this prayer slowly and softly so that you feel the words:

"May I be happy, may I be well, may I be at peace, may I be safe." Then pause and sit quietly. Add additional verses for people you care about. "May _____ be happy, may _____ be well, may _____ be at peace, may _____ be safe." When you are ready, add another verse for someone you feel has injured you. Conclude by affirming, "I offer compassion and my heart responds."

Today I offer compassion to myself and others.

Forgiving

Rejection, betrayal, and humiliation are painful and can cause resentment and thoughts of revenge. The desire to punish, as understandable as it may be, closes off your heart chakra. Then anguish flourishes and inner peace withers. Even though you have been hurt, if you don't practice forgiveness, you pay a high price because forgiveness keeps your heart open, helps you understand human suffering, and reduces your emotional pain. Plus you can forgive the person without excusing, condoning, or even understanding what happened. One way to forgive is by doing a meditative practice on air, the element of the heart chakra. Air permeates all life, from your lungs to the sky overhead. Light, invisible, and free as the wind, air is necessary for life. Similarly, heart energy is expansive and necessary for human life.

For this practice, sit meditatively. Consider the person you want to forgive (possibly even yourself) and what you want to forgive him or her for. Close your eyes and breathe into and out of your heart for a few minutes, feeling the movement of air. When you are ready, focus on your heart and visualize the person you want to forgive. Breathe in and say, "I forgive," then breathe out and say, "I release." Conclude by affirming, "I breathe in forgiveness and breathe out suffering."

Today I practice forgiveness,
beginning with this breath.

A Supportive Atmosphere

Your heart is responsive to its surroundings, including what the people you associate with say, as well as your own thoughts. Keeping your heart open is easier when you are around people whose words reflect understanding, optimism, and reverence for life. Therefore, seek out unpretentious people who smile often and say uplifting things. Get to know them. Ask what matters to them and share what matters to you. This mutual respect and friendship will buffer you from pessimism and help you be kind. Perhaps even more importantly, learn to be a good friend to yourself. Get off your case and have faith that the future is bright. Calm doubts and insecurities when they arise, refocusing on "It will be okay" and "My heart knows best" thoughts. Feel as though someone on the inside is holding your hand

and encouraging you along. The following is a practice of creating a group of people, animals, and ideas inside yourself that you can call upon.

To practice, make two columns in your journal. In the first column, create your internal support system. List names or post pictures of individuals and animals, living or deceased, who motivate and inspire you. In the second column, write words of wisdom, including quotes and scriptures that lift you up. Conclude by affirming, "I surround myself with people and ideas that keep my heart open."

Today I cultivate a supportive atmosphere.

Bowing in Gratitude

Being thankful for your joys and your sorrows helps you appreciate how sacred and transient human life is. Gratitude is a gentle rain that soaks the parched soil of your mind so flowers of wisdom and love of life can grow. Gratitude embraces grief with the understanding that something irreplaceable has taken new form. Do not be alone with your anguish or with your joy. Give each of them to gratitude so you can honor what you have received and what you have learned. It is beneficial to give thanks for just about everything but truly transformational to give thanks for insights into how incredibly precious life is, how it constantly changes, and how interconnected joy and sorrow are. Gratitude, one of the spiritual energies of the heart, is easy to access, as this practice shows.

To practice, sit meditatively. Breathe into and out from the bottom of your heart. Then, inhaling, stretch your arms out wide from your shoulders. Feel your chest open. Exhaling, cross your hands over your heart. Stretching your arms out, say, "I am grateful for…," and as you place your hands over your heart, say what you are grateful for. Repeat many times, giving gratitude for the mundane, the profound, and lessons learned. When finished, place both hands over your heart and bow. Conclude by affirming, "I have gratitude."

Today I bow in gratitude.

Loving Touch

When your heart opens, you want to touch and be touched by others. However, if you were not touched enough or experienced touch that was hurtful, you may avoid touching or tense up around it. Touch may feel uncomfortable, or you may think that most touch is insincere or harsh. This does not mean that touch is not for you; it means that you have some healing to do before you can enjoy it. Not surprisingly, touch is the sense associated with your heart chakra. Touch from the heart is kind, healing, and soothing. Learn to receive tender touch, and you will be able to give loving touch. One way to learn to enjoy safe, respectful touch is to receive professional touch in the form of manicures and massages. Another way to receive touch and open your heart chakra is hugging meditation.

To practice hugging yourself, sit meditatively. Let your body settle and your breath relax. Then, with the tenderness of a sweet grandparent, put your arms around your chest and belly. Rest one hand over your heart. Pat yourself and rock gently if you so desire. Sit in this tender embrace for a while, also hugging any feelings of discomfort. Feel the sincerity of your touch, then release the hug and sit quietly. When ready, visualize giving hugs to your loved ones. Conclude by affirming, "I accept loving touch."

Today I am touched by love.

chapter 6

Throat Chakra

Your throat chakra is the bridge between your heart and mind. When this chakra is not balanced, the voice of your heart is muffled, your creativity stifled, and your authentic communication suppressed. Then your words express unexamined biases and poor impulse control. Later on you may wish that you could take back what you said because such words cause emotional pain and wound relationships. Your communication style ends up being harsh and hurtful, or indirect and flat, which makes it difficult for you to speak honestly, thoughtfully, and from the heart.

The name for this chakra is *Vishuddha*, which translates as "the purification center." Truth and communication are its central themes. Here you learn to take responsibility for what you say, speak up for what you believe in, and express yourself with sensitivity. Here the tendency to speak in half-truths, the need to talk excessively, and other distortions of communication are subdued. Here you become ever more aware of the power of the spoken word.

Your throat chakra is affected by emotional trauma, especially being lied to by people you trust and love. Living in an environment of frequent yelling, excessive criticism, damaging secrets, and authoritarian righteousness can make it difficult for you to trust your own perceptions and speak up for yourself.

An important aspect of purification is examining old beliefs. The element associated with this chakra is limitless space, which makes it easier for you to see your biases and opinions. When your mind is empty of thoughts, it is filled with stillness. This does not mean that your mind is blank; it means thoughts arise in a stillness that continues to be present even when you have thoughts, just as the vast sky is present even when there are clouds. Learn to recognize stillness and you will discover that your mind is as unbounded as the sky. Then you are able to watch thoughts go by like passing clouds and be less pushed and pulled by old ideas and impulses.

Sooner or later you realize, at least to some degree, how much suffering is caused by your undisciplined mind. You also begin to understand that happiness truly comes from within. Gradually you come out from under the spell of unexamined viewpoints and take responsibility for how you interact with others. You discover, through your own experience, that peace results from your learning when to listen, when to speak, and what to say. These discoveries make your voice a welcomed one and inevitably transform your communication with others.

The sense associated with this chakra is hearing. The quality of hearing depends on where you listen from. Listen to others from that place of inner quiet, rather than assuming you know what is going to be spoken, and you will listen deeply. Quiet and tuned in, you can hear others express tender human vulnerability and profound insights. From this place of inner quiet, you can truly hear yourself. You hear the wisdom of your heart, the prejudices of your mind, and your shared humanity with others. These understandings cause your voice to become healing and kind. Your authentic voice comes through, and your words benefit yourself as well as others.

Honoring That Which Purifies

Difficulties, wounds, and attitudes that are unexamined can morph into subtly oppressive beliefs that impair well-being and communication. They become a veil that prevents you from being aware of the deepest longings of your heart. Fortunately, when old subconscious motivations for security, power, and approval are brought up into the light and met with understanding, they lose their power (Keating 2009). Then negative experiences give birth to wisdom. They show you how pain is passed from one generation to the next and how your attitudes and motivations are influenced by past experiences. These important insights alter the way you talk to yourself and others. Your speech becomes more kind. This chakra's energy is akin to a rainstorm that cleanses the land and then dissipates, allowing the sun to shine once again. The first meditation focuses on locating this chakra.

To practice, sit meditatively in a quiet room. Close your eyes, and for a few minutes focus on your breath moving down through your throat as you breathe in, and back up your throat as it goes out. Next, place the first two fingers of one hand in the hollow area of your throat, at the front of the neck. This is the area of your throat chakra. Focus your attention here. When ready, release your hand and sit quietly. Conclude by affirming, "I am open to understanding and transforming my past."

Today I honor the impact of my past.

Accessing Inner Space

Anxiety that makes it difficult to speak up for yourself is often linked to a belief that what you have to say doesn't matter. Some story deep inside about personal insufficiency has a chokehold on your voice. Opening your throat chakra may release the grip of such beliefs and allow you to see them as deceptive carryovers from the past. The element for the throat chakra is space. Space pervades everything, including your mind and the sky. Envision your mind as space, or the sky, and it becomes easier to see anxiety-producing thoughts as clouds passing by. This puts you outside the thoughts, looking in at them, so you can study how they affect you and see their relationship to previous situations. Amazingly, events that led to negative thoughts become learning experiences that touch your heart and change your perspective on life. You feel less damaged as you realize that you are more than what happened and accept yourself as you are.

For this meditation, inspired by Swami Saradananda (2008), sit in a location where you can see the clear sky. Breathe comfortably into your throat and body. Look at the quiet, unmoving, peaceful sky. Close your eyes and imagine your mind as the sky. Experiment with feeling empty and vast. When you are ready, open your eyes. To conclude, affirm, "I feel spaciousness inside myself."

Today I am aware of peaceful space.

The Truth About Guilt

True guilt as an emotion is associated with doing something that your conscience says is morally wrong. You may also feel false guilt, when you are innocent of wrongdoing but believe you caused something bad to happen, such as making someone treat you unjustly. Guilt, whether linked to a previous unwise choice or misguided self-blame, can paralyze your voice. Guilt blocks this chakra. You open your mouth to speak, and your throat becomes constricted, causing you to swallow and say nothing. Intentionally and gently opening this chakra allows you to face the truth about guilt in a way that sets you free. You confess guilt related to misbehavior and reclaim the innocence that underlies false guilt. Blue is associated with this chakra. Blue has a cooling, soothing influence and symbolizes healing, peace of mind, and devotion to spirit. The following meditation helps open this chakra.

To practice, sit meditatively in a quiet location. Close your eyes and focus on your breath. Then direct your attention to your throat area. Relax your throat. Envision the color of the blue sky filling your throat and expanding softly beyond. Focus on this image and allow your throat to feel open and cool for several minutes. Conclude by affirming, "I acknowledge real guilt and release false guilt."

Today I accept the truth about guilt.

Reflecting on Truth

Your voice, an incredibly powerful tool that reveals your motives and desires, is an extension of your inner world. Speech that communicates your deepest aspirations makes life better because speaking about important matters breathes life into them and makes them real. Using your voice for what it is designed for—expressing truth—becomes possible only when you know what really matters to you. The purification process for this chakra includes becoming aware of your innermost yearnings. Inside, you know what you aspire to. However, you can hesitate to look at what you know is true and run away from it. You can also deceive or sabotage yourself with negative thoughts. If you do, you end up wasting your words on conversations of little value. The practice of *manana*, or reflection, reveals your deepest desires, the main obstacles, and the steps you need to take. Reflection also helps you to be discerning—to know which internal voices to listen to and act upon. Therefore, do not hesitate to ask important questions. Risk the journey of discovering.

For this practice, allow time for journaling. Sit meditatively for a few minutes. Then write in response to three questions: What matters most to me? Which old attitudes are in my way? What do I need to do? After journaling, sit quietly. Conclude by affirming, "I want to discover what is most important to me."

Today I am willing to know my truth.

Accepting Responsibility

It is tempting to blame others for your discontent; and it is true that misfortune and cruelty cause pain, change life circumstances, and can be difficult to deal with. Yet blaming others for the state of your inner life is not helpful. It places responsibility for inner peace outside you and breeds fear, jealousy, and resentment. When you lay blame on others, the "it's them, not me" mentality blinds you to your mistakes, prevents you from changing, and diminishes your contentment. Peace decreases as you blame others and increases when you accept responsibility for yourself. It decreases when you focus on negativity and increases when you focus on what is good. The breathing practice of *ujjayi,* or victorious breath, strengthens and unblocks your throat chakra. This practice steadies your mind, creates sound to neutralize negativity, and prevents the rapid breathing associated with frustration.

For this practice, sit meditatively. Open your mouth and exhale, saying "haaa" to hear the sound you will make in victorious breath. Now close your mouth and inhale through your nose, making the same "haaa" sound. Exhale through your nose, sounding "haaa." Continue nostril breathing while making the sound "haaa." Focus on the soothing sound and enjoy the experience of disciplined breathing for a few minutes. Then sit meditatively for several minutes. Conclude by affirming, "I recognize blaming thoughts and accept responsibility for my well-being."

Today I discipline my mind.

Inner Knowing

The still, small voice of inner knowing does not argue or justify—it simply points the way. Because it does not make a fuss, intuitive knowing can be drowned out by the loud sounds of fear, anger, and self-doubt. When it is, you make choices that do not reflect what you truly want or need to do. You do not go wrong when you follow inner knowing. Its journey may not be easy, but it is the way of truth, wisdom, and your heart. Hearing your intuitive voice is easier when the voices of fear, anger, and low self-esteem are subdued. Chanting sacred sounds is a powerful practice that quiets emotional turmoil and attunes you to your higher self. Chanting opens your throat chakra and tones your vocal cords, empowering you to listen to your innermost knowing. The chant *So'ham hamsa,* translated as "That I am, I am that," points to your identity as higher consciousness or an aspect of God.

For this practice, sit meditatively in a quiet space. If you like, hold a rosary, mala, or beads in your hands. Begin softly chanting the words, moving your fingers over one bead with each repetition. Repeat the chant for several minutes. Then silently meditate, gently focusing on your breath. Conclude by affirming, "I am soothed, quiet, and receptive."

Today I listen for the quiet voice within.

Purifying My Voice

Your voice is a powerful instrument. The words you use and the tone of your voice create significant consequences, for better or worse, whether you are talking to yourself or to others. A kind yet honest voice creates a loving atmosphere inside you and between you and others. However, if used to criticize and distort, your voice passes on fear, anger, and despair. When the sanctity of life is foremost in your mind and you pause before speaking, your voice becomes melodious, promotes harmony in your relationships, and soothes emotional pain. Since you express your mind through speech, there is a direct relationship between purifying your mind and using your voice for its highest purpose. Chanting "Om" is a cleansing practice that releases blockages in your throat chakra and focuses your mind on higher consciousness. A droning sound, Om is a sacred incantation that is made up of three sounds: *aaah, oou,* and *mmmm.* When chanting, hold each sound for as long as is comfortable.

For this practice, sit comfortably in a quiet location. Take a couple of deep breaths. Then take a nice breath in and begin softly chanting the sounds of Om. Feel the vibration in your throat. After chanting several rounds, sit in quiet meditation. To conclude, affirm, "I chant the sacred sound so that my voice may be truthful and kind."

Today I tune my voice to be a sacred instrument.

Taking Care of Resentment

Resentment messes up relationships and gets in the way of peace. When resentment runs high, it can be so loud that it is difficult to hear your voice of reason and feel your heart. While angry emotions are part of human experience, when not attended to, they can gain momentum and damage relationships. Intimacy does not arise when you experience ill will, and it is foolish to attempt to resolve grievances in the heat of indignation. Mounting irritation is a signal to take care of your anger before being present to any other relationship. Stop and breathe deeply. Take time out to calm down so you can remember what is important and unblock communication. The yoga pose called lion's breath opens your throat chakra and neutralizes negative energy.

To practice, kneel on the floor and then sit back on your heels. Let your spine be upright. Place your palms firmly against your knees, straighten your arms, and splay your fingers like the claws of a large cat. Breathe in through your nose. Open your mouth wide, stretch your tongue out, look toward your nose, and exhale slowly and forcefully through your mouth, making a loud "ha" sound similar to a lion's roar. Repeat a few times, until you are calmed. Then sit in quiet meditation. Conclude by affirming, "Taking care of resentment helps me take care of relationships."

Today I practice for the sake of my serenity.

The Sound of Silence

It is important to make friends with silence. Doing so helps you know when to talk and when to remain quiet. Silence gives you time to listen deeply to yourself so you can be discerning about what you say and when you say it. You have probably experienced the regret caused by not expressing your truth and the remorse caused by uttering harmful words. Hearing, the sense associated with the throat chakra, includes inner listening. You can listen only when you are not speaking. *Mouna*, or observing silence, is a profound practice that purifies your speech. Silence is a supreme teacher. In silence you literally hear the thoughts that pass through your mind, including deeply entrenched expectations and judgments. Intentional silence subdues impulsive talking and helps you reflect upon your words. Silence also quiets your busy mind and enables you to listen to your heart. Finally, silence is the language of God and the sound of indescribable peace.

To practice observing silence, schedule a period of intentional silence, beginning with one hour. This is a time to be with your inner life and enjoy routine tasks. Refrain from reading, watching television, exercising, and other activities that require an external focus. Gradually increase the amount of time you spend in silence. Conclude your period of silence by affirming, "Being silent helps me truly listen."

Today I make friends with silence.

chapter 7

Third Eye Chakra

The tremendous potential of your mind has to be culti-vated, as the mind cannot maximize its capacities without your active effort and focus. Unless you help it out, the vast capacities of your mind are likely to remain dormant and underdeveloped, because the ability to think deeply and clearly while utilizing intuition takes careful training. As Swami Saraswati stated, "You are trying to harness the energies of the mind" (1984, 95). Opening the third eye chakra helps you train your mind and utilize its potential.

The third eye chakra is located between your eye-brows. Its Sanskrit name, *Agni*, means "to know, to obey, or to follow." Situated in the most recently evolved and uniquely human part of your brain, the frontal lobe, the third eye chakra is in the brain's command center. It has great responsibility: discerning what is true and what is false, controlling your impulses, making decisions, guiding your actions, and being aware of what is going on. To handle these responsibilities, it relies on its capacity for observation, concentration, and decision making.

Opening the third eye involves practices that not only teach you to focus and observe but help you understand what to pay attention to and what to base decisions on. Accordingly, these meditative practices help you quiet your mind and listen deeply so you have access to intuition and important insights.

Certain life experiences can block or disturb your third eye chakra. This was especially true when you were a developing child, as you were highly affected by what went on around you. In addition, living in a toxic environment as an adult can be disruptive to your mind. So, if you were raised in or live in an intimidating environment, you may be highly skilled at scanning the outer environment for signs of danger but less skilled at observing your inner world, including your thoughts. If what you saw didn't match what you were told, you may have only partially developed your capacity to separate truth from falsehood, and if your intuition was invalidated, you may not trust the small, quiet voice of inner knowing.

When Agni is not open, you have little opportunity to confront beliefs that cause you to view the world through the lenses of fixed, narrow perspectives. As a result, you may live under limited or false ideas about what life is truly like. Being under the influence of rigid, life-negating beliefs reduces your access to imagination, including the ability to envision a better future for yourself and others. Such beliefs make seeing the bigger picture next to impossible and put you at risk of setting your standards too low or unachievably high. Also, if you are easily distracted, you may lack discipline and persistence in following through on what matters to you.

The meditative and breathing practices that open Agni are calming, soothing, and easy to perform. Do not be deceived by their simplicity, for they will definitely quiet your mind and help you access inner guidance. Along the way, they will teach you to watch thoughts rather than blindly adhere to them, concentrate on what is most important, become comfortable with inner quiet, and experience profound peace.

Moving Close to Stillness

Wishful thinking, worry, or thoughts that wander all over the place contribute little to your decision-making process. You may be at the mercy of such thoughts when you need to make important decisions, if you do not train your mind against them. Additionally, though it is often wise to consult with others, some decisions are yours alone. Do your research and discuss your options; but in the end learn to trust yourself, because you have to live with your choices. A reliable way to increase your ability to make wise decisions is by taking time to meditate. Meditation shifts your attention away from superficial and psychological matters and into the quiet realm of your mind, which is the home of the still voice within. Even if you do not receive inner guidance while meditating, you are sitting near the seat of wisdom and learning to wait, listen, and trust. In due time, in its own way, wisdom speaks. One practice that helps access stillness in your mind is meditating on a sacred word such as *Om* or *amen*.

To practice, sit meditatively. Silently recite your sacred word. Let your mantra recede when stillness overtakes you, and return to it when thoughts arise. Simply be in silence. Practice for twenty or more minutes. Conclude by affirming, "I sit with stillness."

Today I move closer to stillness.

My Pristine Mind

Looking at life through the lens of beliefs like "You just can't trust people" causes fear, isolation, and loneliness. Fortunately you are not doomed to peering through lenses that rob you of intimacy with others. You can put aside lenses distorted by painful beliefs about people and life to see more clearly how much you need close relationships and how others also need contact. If your mind is like an ocean, thoughts are like small boats and beliefs are powerful ships. Recognizing how big your mind is, including the vast space underneath passing thoughts, helps you get off thought boats. Then you realize that you are the one who sees, not the beliefs you look through. The following meditative visualization inspired by Swami Saradananda (2008) is a way to experience your mind as being as clear as pristine water.

For this practice, sit meditatively. First focus on breathing. Next, visualize your mind, including the area behind your eyebrows, as a clear blue lake. Imagine a brilliant diamond descending through the water and finally coming to rest on the bottom of the lake. Gaze at the diamond for a couple of minutes, then release the image and notice that your mind is clear. Conclude by affirming, "Underneath my thoughts, my mind is still and clear."

Today I notice the spaciousness
beneath my thoughts.

Experiencing Tranquillity

There is little peace in your mind when beliefs like "It has to be this way and only this way" ensnare your attention. These beliefs are like pesky insects that cause tension in your body and frustration in your mind. When rigid thoughts are persistent, they can feel as intrusive and unwanted as mosquitoes and prevent you from getting things accomplished. You can even feel stung by those thoughts, as if you had no choice in the matter. Fortunately, your attention belongs to you, not to your thoughts, and you have a choice. You can intentionally concentrate on something pleasing to release the grip of undesired thoughts. One yogic concentration practice, *tratak,* or "steady gazing," will focus your attention and help your uptight mind become a tranquil mind. *Tratak* trains your attention and soothes your mind, especially when done frequently.

To practice, sit meditatively in a quiet location without a draft. Softly gaze at a lighted candle placed at eye level about arm's length away. Gaze for up to a minute, then close your eyes and envision the flame at the point between your eyebrows for another minute or so. Repeat once or twice, each time holding the image of the glowing flame a little longer in your mind's eye. Conclude by affirming, "My mind is as serene as candlelight."

Today I cultivate a tranquil mind.

Exploring My Clear Mind

Witnessing thoughts helps you realize that thoughts pass through your mind, but they are not your mind. Thoughts come and go, and your vast mind remains. Learn to observe thoughts and you are able to recognize when you are under the influence of attitudes like "Life is just too hard" that discourage and deflate you. When you recognize gloomy thoughts that darken your life and let them pass by rather than holding onto them, your mind feels clear, which causes you to feel well balanced. This gives you enough of a break to consider more optimistic views of the way life is. The following meditation practice releases the hold that pessimistic thoughts have on your attention and enables you to experience your mind as undisturbed, like a clear sky. With repeated practice, you will realize that your mind is so much more than long-believed thoughts.

To practice, sit meditatively. Focus your attention on the point between your eyebrows. Imagine breathing into and out from your third eye. When you notice that your attention has drifted to thoughts, silently whisper, "Thought." Visualize the thought as a cloud passing by in the sky. Then refocus on your third eye. Continue for ten to twenty minutes. Conclude by affirming, "My mind is like a clear sky."

Today my mind is open and clear.

The Way of Truth

Partial truth is as useless as vague directions, or inaccurate directions that tell you to travel east instead of west on the right road. You end up either turning around or not reaching the destination you are searching for. Whole truth, which relies on intellect and intuition, knows what you yearn for and can show you which way to go. Whole truth also requires that the left and right sides of your brain work together in harmony. When the left side—associated with reasoning, objectivity, and positive emotions—is dominant, you tend to be logical. When the right side—associated with mysticism, receptivity, and negative emotions—is dominant, you tend to be creative. When both sides are balanced, you become wise and intuitive. The yoga practice of alternate breathing, *nadi shodhana*, balances your brain hemispheres and helps you access whole truth.

To practice, sit comfortably. With your right hand, press your thumb on your right nostril and breathe in through your left nostril. Then, using your right hand, press your ring and little finger on your left nostril and breathe out through your right nostril. Leave your fingers on your left nostril as you breathe in through the right. Now return to the first position and breathe out through your left nostril. Continue breathing in left, breathing out right, breathing in right, breathing out left. After a few minutes, remove your hand and breathe naturally. Conclude by affirming, "I feel open to the truth."

Today I practice the way of truth.

Approaching Wisdom

Inner knowing may come in a flash or slowly dawn on you. Occasionally you may even think your way into it. However, attempting to force wisdom often leaves you with answers that perpetuate old emotional needs or ways of looking at things. To receive wisdom, approach it with the stillness that comes over you when you enter a sacred place. Ask a sincere question and then wait with a sense of not knowing. When you are as quiet as a child resting on the mother's breast, you enter the inner sanctuary of silence, the home of wisdom. Sooner or later, when you are ready, wisdom will make itself known. The following practice of breath retention will quiet your soul and take you into the domain of wisdom.

To practice, sit meditatively. Do a couple of rounds of alternate-nostril breathing, as in the preceding meditation. Then add a counting pattern of two-eight-four. Inhale to the count of two through your left nostril, hold the breath to the count of eight with both nostrils closed, and breathe out to the count of four from the right nostril. Breathe in for two counts through the right nostril, hold for eight with both nostrils closed, and breathe out for four counts from the left nostril. Repeat. Stay in your comfort zone. Practice for five minutes. Then sit quietly for several minutes. Conclude by affirming, "I open to wisdom."

Today I wait and listen.

Opening to Inner Guidance

If you have experienced a lot of chaos, you may understandably want security. After all, being in a stable environment makes it easier to feel peaceful inside. However, when seeking safety becomes more important than experiencing your potential, you may dismiss inner guidance with thoughts like "No way could I do that." The still voice within, concerned with your continued growth and well-being, can at times take you out of your comfort zone and require that you confront limiting beliefs. At times that small, quiet voice is drowned out by the voice of fear. You need a way to calm your nerves so that you can hear and act on your inner guidance. The breathing practice that follows, *bhramari*, focuses attention on your third eye and settles your nerves, enabling you to accept inner guidance.

To practice, sit comfortably. Bring your hands to your face. Using light pressure, plug your ears with your thumbs, place your index fingers on your eyelids, middle fingers on your nostrils, ring fingers above your upper lip, and little fingers below your lower lip. Focus your attention on your third eye. Breathe in deeply; while exhaling, make a soft humming sound, like a bee. Repeat the breathing pattern several times. Then sit quietly or meditate for a few minutes. Conclude by affirming, "I soothe fear and open myself to guidance."

Today I accept guidance.

Why I Am Here

When the unfortunate behavior of loved ones causes you and others to suffer, you may desire above all else to be a good person who doesn't hurt others. In attempting to be good, you may strive to become like someone else without really discovering your life's purpose. Truly living requires that you learn to live from the inside out, so your life choices can be based on knowing why you are here. The following story of the great Rabbi Zusha points to the importance of being guided by your inner voice of knowing. The rabbi's students gathered at his side as he lay on his deathbed, crying. When asked, "Rabbi, why do you cry?" he said, "I'm afraid when I get to heaven, God is not going to ask, 'Why weren't you more like Moses or Jesus?' I'm afraid that God will ask me why I wasn't more like Zusha. Then what will I say?" Knowing why you are here requires accessing the small, still voice within that meditation gives you access to. So take time to meditate, and take time to ask important questions.

To practice, sit meditatively. Focus your attention between your eyebrows. Imagine breathing into and out from your third eye. After sitting in quiet meditation, ask, "Why am I here?" Then listen. Conclude by affirming, "I want to know my true purpose."

Today I accept that my life matters.

Dedication to My Peaceful Mind

You bathe so that your body will be as healthy and comfortable as possible. Your mind also needs loving attention for it to serve you well and be easy to be close to. If you truly want your mind to be peaceful, perform the meditative practices that open Agni, because inner peace depends on your capacity to witness thoughts, access inner wisdom, concentrate on what matters most, and enjoy stillness. Go to your meditation chair or cushion daily, not just once in a while. Go to your meditation chair or cushion even when a quiet mind eludes you, when answers do not come, or when you see no progress. Go to your meditation chair or cushion even when you do not want to. Solemnly vow to engage in a daily practice. Make your practice inviting, not burdensome. Begin with the practice that you are most attracted to. Sit for five or ten minutes, then gradually lengthen your practice time to thirty minutes. Trust and be faithful to your practice. Benefits of meditation accrue over time.

To dedicate yourself to a daily practice, sit meditatively for several minutes. Then make a vow to practice daily. Conclude by affirming, "I take care of my mind."

Today I dedicate myself to a peaceful mind.

chapter 8

Crown Chakra

Inner peace deepens as the illusion of separateness dissipates and you realize that you are like an individual wave completely indistinguishable from the ocean. The doorway to realizing mystic union with life is the crown chakra, also known as the doorway to God. *Sahasrara*, its Sanskrit name, means "thousandfold" or "infinite," and its symbol, a thousand-petaled white lotus, represents purity and spirituality. When awakened, the crown chakra is said to be like lotus petals opening to brilliant light pouring down from many suns. The elements and emotional pain of the lower chakras give way in the consciousness of this chakra, just as muddy, mighty rivers lose their form when they flow into the ocean.

Like the other chakras, the crown chakra is sensitive to trauma, including abuse by religious leaders, forced religiosity that forbids questioning, or violence that causes you to doubt the spiritual essence of people or the existence of a friendly universe. Such traumas can cause you to feel alone and lost, robbing you of joy and purpose. In the aftermath of trauma, you may turn to status or possessions for meaning, or you may make life be about intellectual prowess and adopt an attitude of philosophical superiority. But when you turn from the sacred, even for understandable reasons, something is missing deep inside.

When you are unaware of your spiritual essence, you may experience ongoing emotional pain. Loneliness, bitterness, fear, and confusion can accompany you through life. Here is the bottom line: your spirit yearns to be happy and peaceful and wants you to recognize your source. Trust and follow this yearning, and sooner or later you will become united as one— body, spirit, and mind together as a wave in the ocean of consciousness.

Meditation is the yogic practice best suited to opening this chakra and experiencing spiritual union. During true meditation, the mind becomes still. Feelings, emotions, and desires are dormant, and you experience a deep inner peace. You sit in the presence of the transcendent, and spirituality becomes a rich inner experience. Only love, light, and clarity remain. In the same way that the night disappears when the sun appears, pleasures, disappointments, and pain fade away in the presence of divine light.

This chakra represents the ultimate goal of yoga, which is uniting with cosmic consciousness, defined by Swami Prabhavananda as "the Godhead, the Reality which underlies this apparent, ephemeral universe" (Prabhavananda and Isherwood 1953, 15). Yoga philosophy teaches that you are a spiritual being becoming aware of your true nature and that you experience lasting fulfillment and peace by embodying the qualities of your spiritual nature in your daily life.

Eternal happiness is found in the realization that you are a living expression of the divine. So do not give up; remain faithful to your spiritual journey. Although the way may be difficult, stay strong and hold on to your aspiration.

Recognizing the Light

Religion that requires blind obedience, is forced upon you, or espouses doctrines that don't seem right to you may turn you away from spiritual life. As a result, you may distrust religion or believe there is nothing beyond the material world. This perspective may work for some time, even though it narrows your vision of life and decreases your awareness of the interconnectedness of all life. Then some crisis or traumatic incident may leave you feeling adrift, inconsolable, and anxious—or perhaps you start to sense that something is missing or your life is touched by someone who inspires you. You begin to seek the spiritual and, in doing so, enter the realm of the crown chakra. Situated at or slightly above the fontanelle, the soft spot at the top of a newborn baby's head, it is called the center of infinite rays because it radiates like the sun. The following practice acknowledges your crown chakra and its energy, the light of consciousness, which is shown as the radiant glow of halos in images of saints.

To practice, sit in meditation for a while. Then bring your awareness to the top of your head. Visualize rays of sunlight streaming down and bathing you. Feel the warmth of luminous white light. To complete, bow and affirm, "I acknowledge my divine light."

Today I bow to the radiant light.

Being Bathed in Light

Believing that spirituality is something you can add on to yourself can generate considerable anxiety. Such beliefs may cause you to vacillate between trying and giving up, while worrying that you are not getting it right. This kind of philosophy traps you in beliefs that prevent you from recognizing that you already are a spiritual being. When you blindly believe something without examination, your world becomes restricted and confined. But when you see your beliefs and release them to the light, you are no longer their captive. Yoga is a process of stripping away, where you examine and surrender all the thoughts and energies that prevent you from experiencing yourself as a being of light. Light dissolves darkness; when you are bathed in light, your sense of being becomes vast. One way to release thoughts to light is a meditation taught by Swami Saradananda (2008) in which you envision brilliant white light permeating your body and mind.

To practice, sit meditatively. Imagine streaming light entering through the crown of your head. Let the light flow down, permeate every cell of your physical body, and dissolve every thought. Envision your entire mind and body being filled with light. Recognize radiance as yourself. Conclude by affirming, "I am a light-filled being."

Today I am bathed in the light of my true self.

Experiencing Stillness

Your mind can become consumed with solving problems and fixing other people. Without your intervention, these thoughts can take over your thinking mind, shrink your world, and reduce your experience of life to what needs to happen. Then you feel tense and experience little joy. There are real concerns in life, and yet, when you are trapped inside a perspective of being overly responsible, you do not know what you can and cannot control. You need a break, a way to get out of your mind-set and into a state of awareness where you are not confined by thoughts. Taking time away from thinking will help you see things more realistically. Beyond your thoughts is infinite consciousness. Give your thoughts to the universe and your mind settles. Then you are alert and conscious, while your mind is as quiet as humanly possible. In this state of stillness, you

Yoga Mind, Peaceful Mind

feel peaceful. This practice of dissolving the elements (Saradananda 2008) is a way to experience stillness in your mind.

To practice, sit meditatively. Imagine land eroding into a river, water being evaporated by the sun, fire dispersing into air, the atmosphere dissolving into space, space being absorbed by the mind, and your mind merging into the infinite. Continue to sit quietly for several minutes. To conclude, affirm, "I experience stillness and I know inner peace."

Today I give my thinking mind a break.

Surrendering to God

Believing you are alone creates extreme anxiety. In reality, you are not alone. You are not intended to go it alone. Accordingly, the main way to relieve the pain of believing that you are a lone soldier—a result of misinformation—is to experience connection. Your body does not live alone; it requires food, shelter, air, and affection. Your mind does not live alone; it interacts with what is happening around it. Your spirit does not live alone; it is like a wave in the ocean of life, and it yearns to be recognized by you. When you are unaware of your spiritual essence, your thinking mind may say that you will know peace when you achieve another accomplishment. However, lasting peace arises when you discover your innate, divine nature. The yoga practice of *isvara pranidhana* means intentionally surrendering your life to God; it involves laying your fears, hopes, and efforts at the feet of the divine. The practice is as simple as reverently saying, "Thy will be done in my life."

For this practice, sit meditatively. Bow forward in a gesture of surrender. Alternatively, kneel down, then bow your head to the floor in an attitude of prostration. Simply pray, "Thy will." Conclude by affirming, "I surrender."

Today I surrender like a wave in the celestial ocean.

Devotion to the Divine

Adhering to "It's dangerous out there" as a life philosophy upsets your body and worries your mind; it dominates and even contaminates your relationship with the divine. Life then narrows to keeping yourself and your loved ones safe. Your prayer life may consist primarily of petitioning an external god for protection. Praying "help me" is a vulnerable and very real aspect of spiritual intimacy; however, much more is available, including friendship and deep love. Your spiritual life is so fundamental that how you relate to the divine determines how you relate to life. When you expand your spirituality to include intimacy with the divine, your anxiety and fearful philosophy will be greatly reduced. You can become aware of higher consciousness as a loving inner presence through worship, or bhakti yoga, where you recognize and appreciate the great worth of the divine. One beautiful practice is reciting the name of the divine during meditation and throughout the day.

For this practice, name your spiritual friend or divine consciousness. Choose a name (such as Beloved, Radiant Spirit, Pure Light, Christ, Buddha, or God) that touches your heart so that saying it is an act of reverence. Sit meditatively and silently recite this name fifty to one hundred times. Then, throughout the day, silently whisper the name as a form of worship. Conclude by affirming, "I draw closer to the divine."

Today I worship the divine.

Surrendering into Stillness

If you feel chronically insecure, you may seek relief in the material world. The belief that money, status, and possessions reduce insecurity is widespread, making materialism seem natural. Food, shelter, and health care are essential, but worshipping material possessions over spirit only bandages insecurity. It temporarily staves off anxiety, but when anxiety rises again, you have to acquire something new. Insecurity begins to resolve when you understand the oneness you share with all life. Even a few experiences of unity are profoundly healing. One way to experience oneness is by practicing a yoga pose called *shavasana*, or corpse pose. In this passive pose, you lie motionless on the floor. Your mind and body become still. This releases emotional pain and allows you to experience the peace of total inactivity (Finger 2005).

For this practice, lie on your back on a carpet or blanket in a quiet room. If desired, place pillows under your head and knees. Let your feet splay open and your arms rest by your sides with your palms face up. Relax your feet and toes, your hands and fingers, your mouth and lips. Rest for a while, between ten and twenty minutes. Conclude by affirming, "I feel peaceful and still."

Today I surrender into stillness.

The Presence of the Sacred

Approaching life with mental certainty is a painful trap. Convictions such as "There is only one way" and "I already know" leave little room for intuition, the insights of others, or the numinous. Philosophical certainty leaves you to make your way through life with mostly unchallenged beliefs. As appealing as it may be to think you have it figured out, such limited knowledge cannot fully comprehend the boundless workings of the universe. Certainty may keep anxiety in check, but it weakens your access to wisdom and a deeply felt interconnectedness. One way to honor your longing to know without collapsing into certitude is reciting "Om" as a prayer. A sacred utterance that represents divine energy, Om begins in emptiness, fills body and mind with vibration, and then returns to stillness. While reciting Om, your sense of personal separateness disappears. Signifying unity, or the undivided oneness of life, Om allows you to experience a universal energy that contains yet extends beyond your body and intellect.

To practice, sit meditatively and contemplate the meaning of Om. Next, chant or silently recite Om for several minutes. Alternatively, chant Om while using a mala or rosary. Then sit peacefully, absorbed in the vibrantly alive yet still energy. To conclude, affirm, "I am filled with sacred energy."

Today I experience the presence of the sacred.

Remembering Who I Am

When your life is mostly focused on your worries, the basic needs of your body, and the events going on around you, you are ensnared. It's as if you were a lotus confined to mud, unable to rise above water. The destiny of the lotus flower is to reach into the light and blossom. So is yours. However, you have free will, and your experience of life is shaped by what you live for. Live as someone who is trying to be spiritual and you will suffer, because you are striving to be something you believe is separate from what you are. Live as a spiritual being immersed in human experience and you will suffer less, because you are able to meet the inevitable problems, anxiety, and despair with compassion and understanding. However, it can take a lot of reminders to keep in mind that you are a sacred being, because busyness and stress can make you forget. One way to reinforce your choice to live as a spiritual being is to take refuge in holy scriptures that reaffirm your spiritual essence. Select a favorite scripture, one that soothes your soul, to read day after day.

To practice, sit meditatively for a few minutes to quiet and center. Next, read and contemplate your scripture. Then sit in quiet absorption. Conclude by affirming, "I accept myself as a spiritual being."

Today I remember who I am.

Intimacy with Stillness

It is natural to want to be finished once and for all with emotional distress and the tendency to fall back into old thoughts and fears. Generally, though, it takes time to release the hold of a lifetime of patterns, including some you may not yet be aware of. Fortunately, a regular practice of meditation provides daily relief, shows you how to rescue yourself when you slip into painful habits, and gradually fills your mind with clarity and peace. After meditating for some time, you will become familiar with stillness. Then stillness can draw you into its arms. You will begin to recognize stillness everywhere, in you and around you. Gradually, stillness will become the center of who you are, the center of all you do. Spending time with stillness will gradually transform your character, relieving anxiety and despair. Focusing on the primary matters of your heart will become easier, and you will begin to lay down your desire for emotional safety, control, and approval. You can hasten the transformation by taking stillness breaks throughout the day, when you stop, feel, and let stillness overtake you.

To practice stillness breaks, set a soothing alarm to chime periodically or ring a bell at regular intervals. Pause in response to the sound. Stop what you are doing, take a couple of breaths, and notice stillness. Conclude by affirming, "Stillness permeates all life."

Today I embrace stillness.

Bibliography

Durgananda, Swami. 2002. *The Heart of Meditation: Pathways to a Deeper Experience.* South Falls, NY: SYDA Foundation.

Finger, Alan. 2005. *Chakra Yoga: Balancing Energy for Physical, Spiritual, and Mental Well-Being.* Boston: Shambhala.

Keating, Father Thomas. 2009. *Centering Prayer Workbook.* Boulder, CO: Sounds True.

Judith, Anodea. 2010. *Chakra Yoga Teaching Manual.* Novato, CA: Sacred Centers.

Osborne, A., ed. 1972. *The Collected Works of Ramana Maharshi.* New Beach, ME: Samuel Weiser.

Prabhavananda, Swami, and Christopher Isherwood. 1953. *How to Know God: The Yoga Aphorisms of Patanjali*. Hollywood, CA: Vedanta Press.

Rama, Swami, Rudolph Ballentine, and Swami Ajaya. 1976. *Yoga and Psychotherapy: The Evolution of Consciousness*. Honesdale, PA: Himalayan International Institute of Yoga Science and Philosophy.

Saradananda, Swami. 2008. *Chakra Meditation: Discover Energy, Creativity, Focus, Love, Communication, Wisdom, and Spirit*. London: Watkins.

Saraswati, Swami. 1984. *Kundalini Tantra*. Munger, Bihar, India: Yoga Publications Trust.

Siegel, Daniel. 2010. *Mindsight: The New Science of Personal Transformation*. New York: Bantam Books.

Mary NurrieStearns, LCSW, RYT, is a psychotherapist and yoga teacher with a counseling practice in Tulsa, OK. She is author of numerous articles on psychospiritual growth, coeditor of the book *Soulful Living*, coauthor of the books *Yoga for Anxiety* and *Yoga for Emotional Trauma*, and has produced DVDs on yoga for anxiety, depression, and emotional trauma. She leads transformational meditation and yoga retreats and teaches seminars across the United States.

Rick NurrieStearns is a meditation teacher, coeditor of the book *Soulful Living*, and coauthor of the books *Yoga for Anxiety* and *Yoga for Emotional Trauma*. For ten years he was the publisher of *Personal Transformation*, a magazine focusing on psychospiritual growth. He has been immersed in consciousness studies and yoga practices for nearly four decades. In 2009 he survived a near-fatal airplane crash that resulted in chronic pain. He credits the practice of meditation with helping him navigate through extreme pain and the journey of recovery.

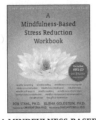
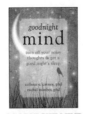
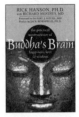
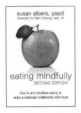
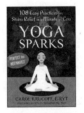
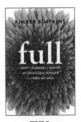
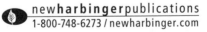